How to

Flip Your Flab— Forever

Harold Hill

with
Irene Burk Harrell
and
Gretchen Black

LOGOS INTERNATIONAL
Plainfield, New Jersey

Scripture references are from the
King James Version of the Bible,
unless noted as NIV (New International Version),
TAB (The Amplified Bible), TEV (Today's English
Version) or TLB (The Living Bible).

Publisher's Preface

My six-foot, four-inch frame could adequately hide moderate overweight. I have never had to diet. When my wife, Viola, started her "slim down" program—and after an insurance examination where I discovered I was fifteen pounds over ideal weight—I remembered Harold Hill's suggestion:

"Dan, let the mind of Christ govern your eating habits."

I began to apply simple rules-of-eating discipline and discovered the Lord's helping ability in providing "food control."

In four months, without starvation or extreme self-denial, I gave away twenty-two pounds and am holding. Yes, it *is* possible to "flip your flab—forever."

Dan Malachuk
Publisher

Contents

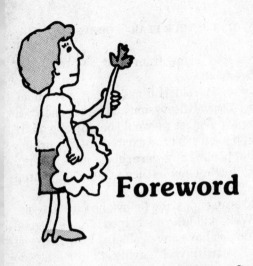

Foreword

Therefore, I urge you, brothers [and sisters], in view of God's mercy, to offer yourselves as living sacrifices, holy and pleasing to God—which is your spiritual worship. Do not conform any longer to the pattern of this world, but be transformed by the renewing of your mind. Then you will be able to test and approve what God's will is—his good, pleasing and perfect will.   (Romans 12:1-2 NIV)

For a number of years I have attempted to fight my ever-increasing enemy. Time and again I would prepare for battle, lettuce leaf serving as my shield and a celery stalk for my sword, determined to conquer. I never realized I was fighting the wrong enemy. You see, I thought my enemy was my girth and of course that came from food so—my mind said—fight the food.

Then one day, Harold Hill and I had just about completed an editorial discussion and he began to tell me about the next project we would be working on. It sounded good but I wasn't too excited about working on another diet book. They were, in my mind, enemy territory, and by now my lettuce leaf was all wilted and my celery stalk was limp.

But Harold is an endearing fellow; he turned to me and said, "Well, kiddo, you helped me real good today. Now do you have any problems I can help you with?" And I heard myself saying, "I certainly do have a problem and it's obvious. It's my fat." There it was, out in the open. Actually it had been out there for quite a while.

Harold didn't even blink. He just said, "Oh, we'll fix that up right now." And he prayed a simple little prayer, asking that my mind would be renewed and that my appetite would be suited to my needs and not my wants.

We hugged and I felt good and forgot about the whole thing.

But shortly after that something happened. For lo, these many years, my clothes bore labels like Lovely Lady and Missey Matron and sizes were two and one-half digits. One day while shopping with a friend, I heard myself declare, "That's the last thing I buy from the fat department."

I found myself involved in a diet program. I had been on diets and in programs before and had "played the game" with counting calories, always attempting to fight the food.

This time I wasn't fighting. I was rejoicing. Every day was victory. And I wasn't having any pity parties. Funny thing, others were having them for me. "How can you not want_____?" they would ask. And I began to realize that my mind was being renewed and my needs were being met and my wants were changing and so was I.

My fighting days are over. My enemy is defeated, not by me, but by Jesus. You see, until my mind began to be renewed, I didn't recognize who my enemy was. Food is not my enemy. Fat is not my enemy. Satan is our enemy.

He is defeated when we purpose in our minds that he is defeated. No celery sword will do him in.

The scripture says we must offer ourselves, we must not conform, we must be transformed by the renewing of our minds and then we will be able to test and approve what God's will is.

Now some sixty pounds lighter, I can share this truth with you.

Until it happens in your head and your heart, it will never happen on your hips—and that is the key to flipping your flab forever.

Viola Malachuk
Plainfield, New Jersey

chapter 1

How This Book Began

Why do people over-eat, over-drink, over-work, over-play . . . over- just about everything?

And is this out-of-balance living a part of the "very good"-ness declared by God in the first chapter of Genesis concerning His creation?

Lots of folks have scores of theories about these things, but theories don't change facts. The excesses keep increasing, especially in the area of flabbitis, as evidenced by the preponderance of pendulous profiles hanging out all over the place. There seems to be a kind of Parkinson's Law for the Paunchy in action—Flab Increases by Astronomical Progression to Overfill the Available Space in the Largest Size You Can Buy.

How come?

Religion calls it gluttony.

Psychology calls it overcompensation.

Skinnies, who don't care about eating in the first place, look down their sanctimonious noses and sneer, "Lack of will power."

Jogging nuts jeer, "It's because you don't get enough exercise."

Even flabbos have their reasons:

"With me, it's a glandular problem."

"Fluid buildup."

"If I don't eat, I get nervous."

"Nobody loves me."

"The kids are driving me crazy. You can't chase a houseful of kids on an empty stomach."

"Those scales must be out of order."

"It's heredity."

"It's my mother-in-law."

"I'm *supposed* to be eating for two."

And there are as many solutions as there are excuses for overweight—or more:

DIETS by the dozens—gimmicky ones and even a number based on good nutrition.

FASTS that eliminate food entirely. If you fast long enough, you can starve yourself into size-six zombiehood. A few weeks more, and you can even eliminate yourself by simple starvation. It's a permanent thing—guaranteed to change your plans for the weekend.

CALORIE COUNTING. But I've noticed that

will turn you into a mathematician sooner than it will make you skinny as a rail. With all the transistorized computers around these days, calorie counting is easier than it used to be, but no more effective in the long haul. As a matter of fact, you may have observed, as I have, that the people in the cafeteria line who have the lowest calorie items sliding along on their trays—naked lettuce, low-cal cottage cheese, black coffee, and lowfat yogurt—are the very ones who have the most inflated spare tires around their middles. Not knowing anything to the contrary, a guy *could* conclude that counting calories is the most fattening thing around.

Diets, fasts, and calorie counting are do-it-yourself solutions. Any flabbo can try them, and probably has at one time or another. Including me. If you go so far as to enlist medical assistance in flipping your flab, you have even more alternatives from which you can choose. Take your pick:

Glandular treatment.

Chemical attack.

Mouth wired shut.

Hypnosis.

Digestive tract bypassed with short-circuit surgery—"at the risk of 5% surgical mortality and 40% post-operative complications," according to *The Harvard Medical School Health Letter*.

You name it, someone can do it for you. They can even cut you open, peel out the globby layers of failure, shorten your skin to fit the new you, sew you up, and send you on your way. Rather expensive, I'm told, but it works—temporarily. If you opt for this last alternative, better ask your scalpel-wielder to install a zipper, because he'll need to peel you out again six months from now.

The trouble with all these solutions is that they all work—temporarily. And keep us from looking at the causes behind the bulges.

If you're like I am—correction, like I *was*—the flab always returns with seven enormous friends after the diet or whatever has ended, merging into the memories of a long line of previous failures. Dozens of "proven methods" have ended up in full-cycle disaster. Inevitably, with the return of the flab, that "loser feeling" comes back, and with it, the attitude that stuffs in another donut, swills another double-malted, reaches for another potato chip dolloped with high-calorie dip, and gulps morosely, "It's just not worth the struggle."

My 6′ 2″ frame permits a lot of latitude in weight variation. I can readily rationalize several pounds above the ideal without too much of a guilt syndrome. "I'm just waterlogged," I say, "been taking in too much salt lately." But when the scales stealthily creak their way up to 215 and threaten *not* to stop there, I'd have to have water on the brain not to get honest with myself and sound the battle cry, "It's got to go!"

Misery sets in for the whole household and anybody else unfortunate enough to get in my path as I deprive myself of bread, potatoes, ice cream, and second helpings of anything except water. I eat cottage cheese until my brain begins to turn to curds and whey. I stow away celery and carrots till my nose twitches like a rabbit.

The pounds melt away—and so do my former friends. But when I've reached my goal, I smile again—and celebrate. How? Ridiculous question! By throwing a party—a real feast—and eating all I want, of course. Everybody rejoices with me—and I'm on my way up the scales again.

But the last time the scales did me dirty, and the dry-cleaners had been shrinking my suits, and the steering wheel had mysteriously inched itself too close to the seat of my car for me to get under the wheel without holding my breath, I got extra honest with myself—and with the Lord.

"It's time for me to flip my flab again," I sighed out loud to Him and to the familiar, friendly double-chinned fellow peering at me from the other side of the mirror. "You and I both know I've been through this thing *so* many times, I'm tired of it. I know I can lose the weight without too much trouble—with Your help, Lord—" (I figured I'd better give Him a little bit of credit) "but the flab knows that as soon as it's gone, I'll do all I can to help it gallop back on me again in record time.

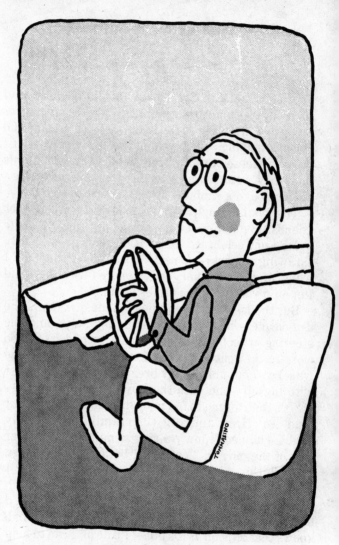

"Help, Lord, my flab won't fit!"

"I've had it with this yo-yo syndrome. It's making me seasick. Is there something *You* can do about it?"

I didn't hear an audible voice—He doesn't speak to me that way very often—but something deep inside, where my gizzard would be if I had one, seemed to say, "Why don't you ask Me for My *permanent* weight-control plan? I have one that will help you flip your flab forever. One that deals with underlying causes instead of surface symptoms. It comes with My highest recommendation. Or would you rather have not because you ask not?"

"Not me, Lord. I'm willing to ask, all right."

I knew He'd answer, too. He'd never failed me yet, in all the times I had tried Him in the past. But I'd never before asked Him for His *permanent* solution, one that would get at the root of my widespread problem. Funny about that, when it was the only sensible thing to do. . . .

And so I asked Him.

"Lord Jesus," I prayed, "please show me why I keep overstuffing myself. Please give me Your permanent answer to this powerful appetite which I'm powerless to control except in the upward direction."

Did He show me?

And how!

Not only did He uncover *why* I never quit eating soon enough, He gave me a perfect method for remedying the situation.

The method was so painless, so simple, I was certain it wouldn't work. How could it? It didn't require any will power. But since I'm a scientist, and a scientist never rejects anything prior to trial, and since the Lord had chalked up such a long record of faithfulness and dependability in my previous dealings with Him, I decided to set an experiment in motion and give His method a try. After all, I had nothing to lose but my flab.

Did it work?

Does rain get things wet?

It worked so perfectly, I knew I'd never have to be a blimpo again. Why, I wouldn't even have a tendency in that direction—as long as I used His plan.

From the moment I turned my excess avoirdupois over to Jesus, and was obedient to follow the clear instructions He gave me, I began to see the numbers on my digital scales count backward: 215, 214, 213, 212, 211 . . . .

At the end of thirty-six weeks, I had lost thirty-six pounds. Without fasting or dieting. No surgery either. No wires about my mandibles. No hypnosis.

How did it happen?

Read on. That's what this book is all about—how I flipped my flab forever, God's way. And how you can do it too.

God bless you as you skinny down for Jesus.

And by the way, if you have an underweight friend, the same approach will bring skinnies back into balance in an upward direction. Unless, of course, other causes need attention from the man with the stethoscope.

"Lord Jesus," I prayed, "please show me why I keep overstuffing myself. Please give me Your permanent answer to this powerful appetite which I'm powerless to control except in the upward direction."

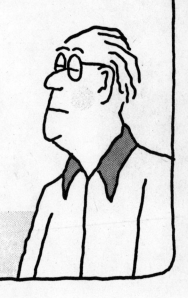

chapter 2

Flabbitis— Facing the Facts

For years I'd had a problem with overweight. I just couldn't say no to all those goodies I met up with on my travels. Oh, I had plenty of Will Power, all right. Trouble is, Will always stuck around just about long enough to hear the Amen after "Lord, we thank You for this food." Then Will vamoosed to a far country and wasn't heard from again until the temptation had vanished—inside me. Will couldn't seem to hang around long enough for victory to set in.

I'd learned to take care of my conscience the first time the goodies were passed. My initial "No thanks" salved my conscience, and it didn't deprive my bloated belly of a thing. The hostess could always be counted on to pass the goodies one more time, cooing, "Oh, Mr. Hill, won't you have just one teensy, tiny

11

bite?"

When she said that, it didn't matter if she was only 4′ 2′′ in platform wedges and weighed a scant seventy pounds dressed for a blizzard—with a backpack—I'd act like she had twisted my arm clean out of its socket.

"Well, I really shouldn't—doctor's orders, you know—but it looks so good—"

A fellow has to flatter his hostess—it's only good manners. And blaming my doctor instead of my tailor, who'd warned me he couldn't let my suits out another fraction of a centimeter, helped my public image immeasurably, I figured. Anyhow, I'd say, "I'll try a little—just this once," but inside I'd be praying she'd give me the biggest piece on the plate.

I don't know whether anyone except my wife ever noticed it or not, but after trying "a little, just this once," I never stopped stuffing it down until the cake plate, pie pan, cookie platter, or what-have-you was as vacant as a swimming pool parking lot in midwinter. And it showed, increasingly, all over me.

Have you been there too, down Gluttony Trail?

Delicious, isn't it? Until you get on the scales the next morning, and the morning after that.

Well, all good things must come to an end, some philosopher said. And fortunately, things that are bad for us can come to an end too. The Lord uses all sorts of ways to get our attention about it. He reached me with a broken rib.

12

I won't go into how I happened to break my rib—there are plenty of ways you can do the same thing, and I don't recommend one above the other. Suffice it to say that a broken rib *can* hurt bad enough to call for the attention of the man in the white coat. The one I went to see held my x-ray up to the light, squinted through his bifocals, and announced, "Broken rib, all right. Ventral fracture adjacent to articulation with the third costal cartilage at the sternum—"

While he reeled out the Latin, I wondered what kind of cast he'd have to put on me for something that sounded so serious. I had visions of a concrete pajama extending from my Adam's apple to my bulging beltline and figured I'd have a perfectly good excuse to look like a stuffed shirt for a while.

"Nothing as bad as all that," the medico chuckled. "A simple elasticized er-uh 'brace' with a few bones for stability will serve very well."

He dragged a vaguely familiar looking flesh-colored garment out of a hospital-white box and trussed it snugly around me, tying some strings in the back where I couldn't get to them.

"There," he pronounced, "that ought to do the trick. It will give you the support you need while that rib is healing."

As I was leaving his office, the receptionist handed me a bill. When I glanced at the bottom line, I was tempted to have a heart attack on the spot, but decided instead I could probably unload the brace at a pawnshop for a small fortune when I finished with it and declare the balance of the investment as a capital loss on my income tax.

"Special surgical garments are sky-high these days—just like everything else," I muttered to no one in particular as I opened the door to go down the hallway. The receptionist smiled, a little too broadly, but she didn't say anything. She seemed extra happy about something though, and I wished her a good day.

As soon as I hit the parking lot, I heard an explosion of riotous laughter in the building behind me, but the walls didn't fall, and I forgot all about it—until the next morning.

The doc had told me to wear the brace twenty-three and three-quarters hours a day—time out for just one quick shower.

I didn't sleep too well that night. That shoe-laced contraption didn't just hug me too tight, it pinched like crazy every time I moved. I could hardly praise the Lord loud enough to drown out my ouches. The pain of a broken rib was like a picnic without ants in comparison.

When it was finally morning, I headed for the shower almost before I had both eyes unglued. Getting out of the flesh-colored cage took some doing, but I made it after innumerable Houdini contortions to get all the laces untied behind my back, nearly spraining both shoulders in the process. *After* it was off, I spotted the hooks on the side that would have simplified the operation, but at least I was out of the thing and could breathe again.

The shower was like heaven, and I made it a long one. For a while, I was afraid there were going to be permanent-press pleats in my folded-over layers of flab. Eventually though, the wrinkles ironed out, the hot water turned cold, and I had a choice—keep standing there and freeze to death or get back into my surgical garment. Since I've never been overly fond of Eskimo climate, I turned off the water, toweled off the icicles, and nerved myself for the ordeal of re-entry into the Chinese torture chamber. No, I'd never been to China, but I had heard about such things.

Pulling Fleshy down from the towel rack where I had slung her, I noticed a sizable label sticking prominently from one of the whale-boned seams. I could read it without my glasses:

GIRDLE. FEMALE. SIZE: X-LARGE.

The nerve of that quack! Can you imagine a guy's own doctor doing such a thing to him?

Support or no support, I wouldn't be caught dead wearing *that* thing again!

Besides being embarrassed and mad, I was secretly disappointed. During the years of my gradually increasing girth, I'd wondered if one of those things my wife wore (so *that's* why it had looked so familiar!) would make me look trim when my jacket was off and my shirt tucked in. I'd just learned, the hard way, that the fool thing would not only kill you with torture, it wouldn't hide the flab.

Oh, it skinnied me down in places, all right, but the squeezed flab squirted out in a little roll up around the top and down around the bottom, giving me roughly the shape of—

Well, I'll leave my shape to your imagination, but nobody was about to nominate me for Mr. Perfect Physique for the Year. Not even for Runner-Up. Enough said.

Then and there I came eyeball to eyeball with the awful truth every plumpie has to face sooner or later:

You can't hide flab. Just like the truth, flab will out.

I never took my surgical garment to a pawnshop after all—never even declared it on my income tax. Instead, on a moonless night, when no one was looking, I did the only sensible thing. After all the neighborhood dogs were asleep, I tiptoed outside with a brown paper bag and stashed it under the clanking lid of the galvanized container behind our neighbor's garage. No, not the neighbor next door, one half-a-dozen houses down the street.

That was the end of my thinking I could ever hide my flab. It had to be faced, head-on.

Chapter 3

There's No Such Thing as Overeating!

Facing flab is hard on the human ego. The natural tendency among us flabbos, once we have faced our flab instead of denying it, once we've learned that we can't hide it, is to rationalize and make excuses for how it got stuck on our frame in the first place.

A chubby chum of my acquaintance told me one day, "Yes, I know I'm too fat, but I don't know why. It must be my metabolism, because I certainly don't eat that much. Why, I eat like a bird."

It sounded like a pretty good excuse, and I wondered if it would work for me. But unfortunately, I already knew better. I had watched a bird at work one day—a little chickadee at the feeder outside our kitchen window.

Amazing! He never quit! There was no way that

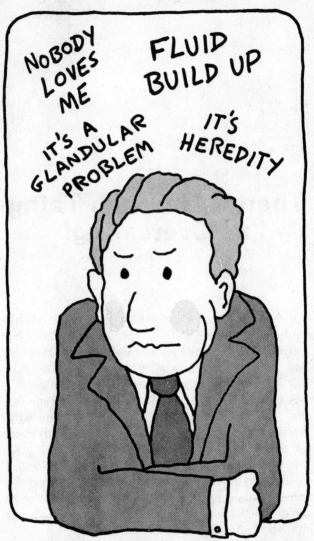

"They all . . . began to make excuse" (Luke 14:18).

tiny creature could eat so much and not be bigger than the Graf Zeppelin in two months' time—unless birds were different from folks and could afford to eat more in proportion to their size without being permanently grounded.

Whatever the reason, it had to be that eating like a bird—a grain of seed or one bug at a time, constantly, without stopping—was one of the biggest no-nos around for folks with tendencies toward pendulous profiles. Only a bird-brained flabbo would mouth the excuse, "I eat like a bird." It was plainly not for me.

Then I thought of the gal who faced her flab without trying to get out of it. Everybody thought she was such a cheerful chubby, such a joyful Jill.

"Yes, I know I'm too fat, and I know why," she grinned behind her oversized dark glasses as she opened a sweet-smelling, grease-spotted white box from the bakery. "I just happen to love to eat, and I don't mind the consequences, so why should you? I'm perfectly healthy—and happy—so lay off!" Then, to show she had no hard feelings, she purred, "Here, have one of my chocolate-frosted cream puffs."

Lots of people—including me—fell for Jill's philosophy and for her cream puffs. We even used her cheery roly-poly-ness as justification for our own. All of us lardos took great satisfaction in pointing in her direction and boasting, "Well, at least I'm not that bad!"

We were really shook up when we read the secret

unveiled in Jill's memoirs, discovered after her untimely do-it-yourself departure from planet earth:

"Sure, I laughed a lot about my size—in public. And I pretended it was okay—in public. But Mr. Lincoln was right when he said you can't fool all of the people all of the time, because I never fooled me. That's why the big dark glasses—to hide my red eyes. When I was rolling with laughter on the outside, I was sobbing real tears on the inside. They spilled over whenever I was alone with the real me. And when I won the all-expense-paid trip for being the most cheerful employee at the plant, I wound up staying in a motel room with twin-sized beds. It was humiliating enough to have to shove them together, but then I went to take a bath, and the bathroom had wall-to-wall mirrors, and—"

Flab's no fun to the one who wears it, no matter what we say. Flab's always a problem, especially when it's on us.

After Jill's funeral, I tried to blame the Lord.

"After all," I argued, "didn't You declare that all parts of Your creation—including our appetites—were very good there in the beginning of things? Didn't You say that Adam and Eve could freely eat of the trees of the Garden of Eden except one? Wouldn't that *have* to mean that us Jacks and Jills could eat all we want? That our appetites would properly regulate our grocery intake?"

I thought I had Him backed into a corner with my

logic, and that I had made out a pretty good case against Him, proving that my flab was all God's fault.

"You're partly right, Hill," He let me know. "In the very beginning, when Adam and Eve were still following My directives—"

Then He sent me back for a quick review of the Garden of Eden history as Moses had written it in the Book of Genesis.

I saw that everything *was* heavenly in paradise in the beginning. There was no flab, no dieting, no calorie-consciousness. And this idyllic state of affairs lasted as long as Adam and his spouse chose to do God's thing, being obedient to the one prohibition He gave them—not to eat of the fruit of the tree of the knowledge of good and evil.

Adam didn't need to know the difference between good and evil in those days, because there was no evil. Everything *was* very good, just as God said, including human appetites and the amount of padding on human torsos.

But then the deceiver came into the picture—Old Slue Foot—suggesting there was something better than perfection as God had planned it.

"If you'll just eat the no-no fruit, you'll be as wise as God," he said.

What an appeal to the ego! No wonder Eve couldn't turn it down. She fell for Slue Foot's angle—hook, line, and sinker. And talked her hubby into sinking along with her.

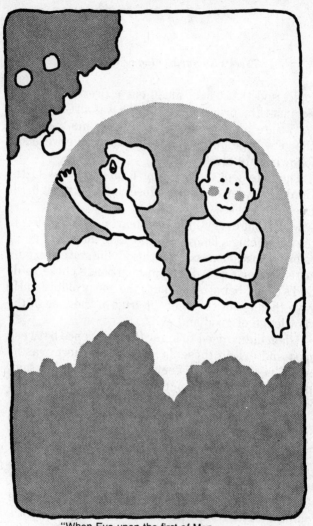

"When Eve upon the first of Men
The apple press'd with specious cant,
Oh! what a thousand pities then
That Adam was not Adamant!" (Thomas Hood)

Things changed in Eden Gardens after that. When Adam and Eve fell, they dragged the whole human race and all the rest of creation down along with them. Thorns and thistles began to grow on the earth, and fear replaced the perfect fellowship man had enjoyed with God. Everything became unbalanced—including human appetites.

So my flab wasn't God's fault—it was the fault of Adam and Eve! Blaming them made me feel better, but it didn't shrink my flab a single inch. As a matter of fact, blaming them was as good an excuse for a pity party as I'd had in a long time. And downing martyr pills and slurping sorry soup while I plotted how I could get even with them probably added a few more inches to my middle.

It took a long time for me to realize it, but when my belt ran out of room for punching new holes, I was finally ready to stop reacting and blaming and to listen long enough to hear what the Lord had to say about it.

"I am the same yesterday, today, and forever," the Word told me, "and like Adam and Eve, *you* can choose to eat of the tree of life—trusting Me, obeying Me—and enjoy the blessings of eternal life right now. Or—" something in His tone of voice made the alternative sound like something definitely second best—"you can keep on with your head-trip, eating of the tree of the knowledge of good and evil, trying to figure everything out for yourself instead of taking

23

My Word for it."

It hadn't occurred to me that I had been gorging myself on the wrong tree and that's why I was getting into such bad shape with all that overeating. . . .

But wait a minute!

A powerful thought came at me from somewhere, a thought that blew my mind because it was so contrary to what I and other flabbos had always believed. The thought was in words that went like this:

"There is no such thing as overeating."

"No such thing as overeating?" I wondered if I'd heard correctly and grabbed the spare tire around my middle to make sure it was still there.

"No such thing as overeating." There it was, a final, for-certain pronouncement. "No such thing as overeating."

I accepted it as truth, against all the reasoning of my educated idiot box, but I had to ask Him one question.

"Lord, I'll accept that from You, that there's no such thing as overeating, but if it's true, then please tell me where *this* comes from." My hands wiggled the roll of flab that was such a prominent fact on my figure. My ears shot up an antenna, listening. And as I waited on the Lord, the understanding came.

"Hill, there's no such thing as overeating. Your flab comes from feeding the wrong part of you. It's a symptom that your appetites are out of balance. Whenever you're hungry, you think your stomach needs groceries, and so you belt them down. But that's not always where the need is. Sometimes your stomach *is* hungry, and needs to be fed, but not as often as you think. Judging from the size of that flab in your hands—" I let go of it then, "your stomach could feed on stored fat for several months without any harm done. But some parts of you are literally starving to death."

"Wait a minute now," I interrupted. "You say my stomach isn't hungry, but some other part of me is starving to death?" It didn't make sense. What other part of me could possibly be hungry? Maybe I needed to take a course in anatomy to grab what He was getting at.

"Lord, You'll have to break this down into kindergarten language if You want me to understand it," I told Him. "I feel like I'm way out in left field somewhere."

One of the things I like about the Lord is that when I ask Him to make it simple for me, He does. And He got through to me with some important truths I'd been ignoring in my long and losing battle with the bulge. They came to me in as simple a form as Pablum for a baby.

chapter 4

Flip Your Flab— By Eating for Three!

"No such thing as overeating. That's a real mind-blower, Lord. And I'm here now just waiting for You to explain it. Seems contrary to the evidence of my senses, with all the distended torsos I see hanging out all over. How can that idea possibly have come from You?"

When I ask Him a question, I expect an answer, and I'm never disappointed. Especially because His answers are so much better than anything I could dream up on my own. This time was no exception.

First, I'm going to give you the shortened version of what He told me, because I know you're eager to get going with flipping your flab forever without further delay. Later, I'll fill you in on important details.

The first thing He showed me is that God looks at us as total persons, whole ones, not as fragmented beings. And He has designed the total person with natural, necessary appetites. These appetites can be broken down into three types. No, Brother Broadbottom, not for mashed potatoes, ice cream, and lobster with drawn butter—

The three types of appetites are related to the kinds of persons we become when we are born again. (You can read all about this necessary step to full creaturehood in my *How to Live Like a King's Kid*, available at your Christian bookstore.)

King's kids, those who have been born again by receiving Jesus, are three-part people—spirit, soul, and body. As someone has put it, man *is* a spirit, he *has* a soul, and he *lives in* a body.

Our spirits have appetites for the things of God. King's kids' spirits feed on *The Manufacturer's Handbook*, which is God's Word in written form, and on the Bread of Life, who is Jesus, the Word made flesh. Our spirits are also nourished by prayer—when we talk to God and listen to Him—by praising and worshiping God, by giving Him thanks in all things, by rejoicing in all He sends our way, by obedience to His laws, by ministering His love to others. . . .

Our souls have appetites, too, our souls being the mind and emotions, the "feeling" part of our existence. Just as we can feed our physical bodies a good diet or a bad one, junk foods or wholesome, nourishing ones, so we can feed our souls what will make them grow in the right direction, becoming more and more at home with God, or we can feed them filth, grumbling, pity parties, and the garbage that spews out of secular TV, fitting our souls for a down-the-tube destination in the final windup.

Our bodies' appetites are so well known to us, we are careful to feed them three squares a day and as many snacks in-between-times as we can arrange.

Three-part persons, three-part appetites. And when everything is in balance, with each of the appetites being appropriately taken care of, health, well-being, joy, usefulness, prosperity, and everything else good can be expected to result. But when any of these appetites is neglected or short-changed, or when any one of them is fed garbage, look out!

Here's an illustration of what happens when the spirit's appetite is not fed with what the spirit needs:

Paula Procrastinator put off her Bible reading for a week.

"I just didn't have time to get around to it," she explained. "No, I didn't have time to really pray either." And of course she didn't get to attend church services on Sunday morning, because she had company for the weekend and everybody slept in. After all, they'd been up late the night before—

Sunday afternoon, after the company left, things

got partially back to normal, but not completely. Because Paula had starved her spirit for a week, its cries to be fed were kind of weak, easy to ignore. And when she felt that "I'm hungry!" inner restlessness, she naturally thought it was her stomach crying for attention.

"I shouldn't *be* hungry, after that big dinner we had," she told her husband, "but I feel like I'm simply starving to death. I'm absolutely famished for something different and delicious, something really good to eat."

Mousey Morris didn't feel like an argument, so he took her out to supper at the most lavish establishment in town, blowing the budget for a month. Afterward, Paula didn't understand why she was still not satisfied. The food had been good enough, but—well, it just didn't hit the spot.

If she had known where the hunger was coming from, she could have gone to the prayer meeting at church instead of to the restaurant. Her spiritual appetite would have been satisfied and the scales wouldn't have told a sad story when she got on them the next morning.

Starving our spirits can lead to overloading our bodies with fat-building calories. And keeping our spirits well fed can lead to good health, no unhealthy craving for excess physical food, no overweight—and long life. Do you want Bible for it? Try this bit from Exodus:

> *Worship the Lord your God* (that would feed
> your spirit, wouldn't it?) *and his blessing
> will be on your food and water* (food that He
> had blessed for your intake wouldn't make
> you sick with excess flab, would it?). *I will
> take away sickness from among you*
> (overweight is reported to be one of the
> most widespread sicknesses in America
> today). . . . *I will give you a full life span*
> (no premature deaths from high blood
> pressure, heart attacks, do-it-yourself
> destruction, or other ailments caused by
> overweight). (Exodus 23:25-26 NIV)

As far as promises go—and God's promises are
good for eternity—that's a pretty all-encompassing
one. Benefits guaranteed—if you keep on worshiping
the Lord your God, an action which feeds your spirit
abundantly.

How about soul hungers? Are they ever
transferred to the physical realm, sending a King's
kid scurrying for groceries when he ought to be
feeding some other part of him? Of course! Haven't
you noticed how often the frustrations of the soul
send folks rushing to the refrigerator or the ice cream
parlor for comfort? Look at some of the examples I've
observed—all in the lives of other people, of course:

Big Bertha chomps her way through a whole box of

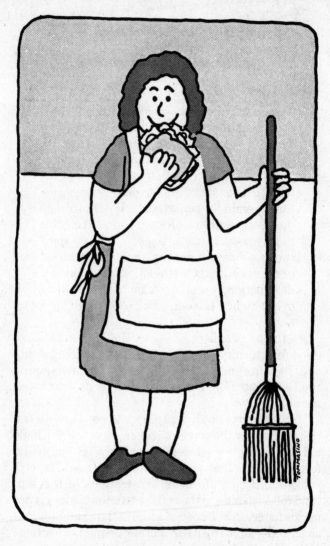

Fight frustration with faith, not food.

chocolates because she has unruly children.

Pudgy Percival belts a few extra beers on his way home from work because the boss blamed him for not getting the coveted contract. It wasn't Percy's fault, of course, but he was afraid he'd lose the job over it anyway.

Acned Agatha, an unpopular teenager, orders a double chocolate malt to comfort herself because she doesn't have a date for the prom.

Sloppy Sylvester snitches an extra handful of butterscotch brownies because mama won't let him play outside until he's cleaned his room.

Girthy Grandma sits down to half a homemade pie a la mode because the neighbors' dog tore up her tulip patch.

Any disappointment will do. Any anxiety will work. Flabbos never have to look far to justify a pity party with refreshments. And I've never yet attended a pity party where the refreshments were skim milk, carrot sticks, and celery curls. They're always something exceedingly fattening. The more forbidding the calorie count, the more appealing the food to the flabbo with hurt feelings, worry warts, and unrejoicing innards.

So often, our flabbitis stems from wrong reactions to life's adversities instead of positive responses to them. Instead of following the directions in the New Testament and rejoicing because we know God is working for our good in all things, we brood everything that's less than perfect into a real down-the-drain catastrophe. Our souls are crying for the fruit of the Spirit to be manifested in the midst of the circumstance, but we feed our bodies groceries of every description in an attempt to satisfy ourselves. It can't work, and it doesn't.

Did you recognize yourself anywhere in the case histories already cited? No? Well, let's add a few more so you'll know you're included. Try these on for size.

Have you ever stuffed your gullet because

• someone hurt your feelings? (A piece of pie will help?)

• you were bored? (A brown sugar sandwich slathered with butter will liven up your life?)

• you let your mind be captivated by gloppy advertisements in magazines or subliminal programming on the boob tube and rushed right out to consume "goonies" you'd never heard of before?

• an expected check failed to arrive in the mail? (Three raw frankfurters will improve your bank balance?)

• you went shopping for a new dress and the rear-view mirror reflected a triple-wide you? (A cup of hot chocolate—with marshmallows and buttered toast—will head your derriere in the *right* direction?)

• the front yard needs mowing, the house needs paint, and two shutters are hanging by one hinge? (Three heaping tablespoons of peanut butter out of the jar will correct the scene?)

• the TV tube is on the blink and the repairmen are out for the week? (A whole tube of artificial potato chips will fix it maybe?)

• you're tired and talk yourself into more calories for energy when the real problem is that you're too fat already? (A whole can of cashews?!)

• your auto insurance isn't going to pay for that bent fender? (You head for the cookie jar as if it was a do-it-yourself repair kit?)

• your kid flunked science? (Two sausages left from breakfast will turn the whole family into Einsteins?)

• your kid is late coming home from football practice and you're worried he might have had an accident? (Before he turns the knob, safe and sound, you've devoured half a box of saltines and a whole pound of cheddar cheese?)

Now do you feel included?
Don't call these things overeating. That doesn't

help, and technically it's not true. You needed feeding all right, but it was your soul that needed satisfaction, not your stomach. The overweight sad sack is taking into his system the required sum of nourishment, but it's all concentrated in one dimension, the physical, and should be spread out in three dimensions for best results.

Up to now, where most flabbos have gone wrong is that they've tried to treat the symptoms instead of the causes. Treating symptoms is seldom effective in the long run. And trying to make an appetite behave results in multiplied frustration. Self-imposed diets and fasts almost guarantee return of the flab in record-setting time. Self-denial breeds compulsion. Want proof?

Look at Eve. What whetted her appetite? Telling her that the no-no-fruit was out of bounds. That naturally increased its desirability. The same tendency is in all of us. Tell me that Drāno is bad for Homo sapiens and I'll start planning a Drāno "trip." Can't help it—that's the way I'm made. Tell me that my excess flab will positively shorten my life by X number of years, and I'll order a second helping of the most calorie-laden banana split on the menu.

But isn't there a way out?

Of course there is. Didn't you ever read, "But God is faithful, who will not suffer you to be tempted above that ye are able; but will with the temptation also make a way to escape" (1 Corinthians 10:13)?

The remedy is wholeness. A *whole* package that will flip the flab comfortably with no adverse side effects—physical, mental, or spiritual. When the natural God-given appetites are distributed properly into the three channels He intended, each channel being nourished instead of all the intake being glopped into the food frequency, unhealthy cravings for body food simply disappear.

That proper spiritual food would reduce excess cravings for body input I knew from experience. I had never even *thought* about being hungry for ordinary groceries in the midst of a really juicy prayer meeting or Bible study, no matter how long it lasted. God had said that would be the case: "Thou wilt keep him in perfect peace [no way-out cravings for anything] whose mind is stayed on thee" (Isaiah 26:3).

He'd also said that feeding the soul what its appetite called for instead of reacting in all the pagan ways would be beneficial.

The scripture for that is one I've quoted most often in my travels around the country. Funny I hadn't noticed before what it had to say about overweight. The scripture comes from John's third letter, and it goes like this:

> Beloved, *I wish above all things* (that's a pretty big emphasis, isn't it?) *that thou mayest prosper and be in health* (no

overweight problem where health is), *even as thy soul prospereth.* (3 John 1:2)

Looks to me as if the Manufacturer Himself is saying plainly that if we will keep our souls prosperous by doing what is good for them, feeding them a right diet, He'll throw in a guarantee of perfect weight as a fringe benefit.

But Lord, what should I feed my soul—the mind, emotions, and feeling part of me that so often sends me to the coffeeshop for comfort? Somehow I didn't think the soul food at the supermarket—blackeyed peas, turnip greens, spare ribs, and cornbread fixings—was what He had in mind here.

Instead, the word *obedience* seemed to come through loud and clear.

"Obedience to what, Lord?" I thought of asking Him, but before I could ask, the answer came directly from the words of Jesus: "Man shall not live by bread alone, but by every word that proceedeth out of the mouth of God" (Matthew 4:4).

Somehow, in that verse, He was saying to me that I was to feed my soul with obedience to everything He had said! That was a bundle! Some of the first things that ran through my mind were forgiveness, patience, love, rejoicing, thanksgiving, meditating on His Word, setting my mind on things above, not being conformed to this world, having the mind of Christ in me, praying without ceasing, being His witness, coveting to prophesy. . . .

In other words, if I would do everything He told me to do, my soul would prosper beyond my highest expectations, and my body would fall in line. Pity parties, holding grudges, taking martyr pills, complaining, being fearful, grumbling—all those things would be gone forever from my life. Never again would I be tempted to be a glutton because my feelings were hurt or I was disappointed in something or somebody.

"Lord, that sounds like living in high victory!" I told Him. "High victory all the time!"

The impression I got was that Someone was saying, "Right on! Right on!"

I decided to check it out with some of the examples I'd just cited of other folks heading for the grocery table when life handed them something other than a bowl of cherries.

Big Bertha chomping chocolates because of unruly children should have resorted to obedience to bringing them up in the way they should go.

Pudgy Percy swilling sludge in an effort to ward off fear of firing should have prayed for the one who did him wrong and given thanks for the very circumstance in which he found himself. Perfect love—Jesus inside him—could have turned imminent disaster into present victory.

Acned Agatha trying to drown her disappointment in the depths of a double chocolate malt should have

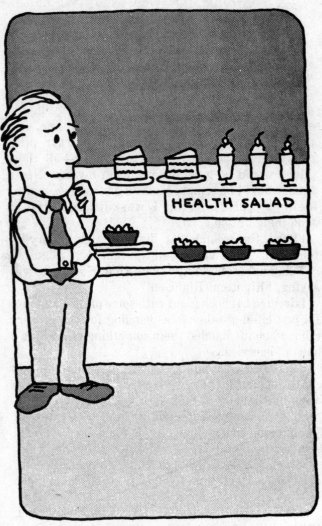

"I will not choose what many men desire" (William Shakespeare).

rejoiced that God loved her enough to send His Son to die for her. The prospect of the smoothest earthly date with a gawky kid would pale in comparison.

Sloppy Sylvester? That's an easy one, Lord. He should have prospered his soul by obedience to the commandment that requires him to honor his mother—and to obey his parents.

Girthy Grandma? She's old enough to know better than to hold a grudge against anybody, tulips or no tulips. Forgiving the neighbor—and the dog—could have filled her with such sweetness that she wouldn't have wanted the pie and ice cream.

It certainly was easy for me to see where Bertha, Percy, Aggie, Grandma, and the others could have mended their ways, but I got the impression I wasn't just to look at *them*—

"When's the last time *you* raided the refrigerator on account of a disappointment or a worry, Hill?" I hung my head, because it was just yesterday. "And did the extra physical food satisfy you?"

"No, Lord. It didn't even taste good. Gave me indigestion to boot. And a bad conscience."

"Do you see what you *could* have done instead—to prosper your soul?"

It was plain as my paunch. My flabbitis *was* a symptom of my out-of-balance appetite.

"Yes, Lord, I see it. I'm to live by every word that comes out of Your mouth instead of stuffing so much garbage into mine. And Lord, already I can see that will make a difference in my life. I *have* been feeding the wrong part of me, all along, but I'll know better now. I'll try obedience first, next time. And I have a hunch it will satisfy."

I was ready to sum it all up for myself, out loud, so He could check me if I didn't have it all straight:

1) I am a three-part person—spirit, soul, and body.

2) Every part of me has an appetite that needs to be fed.

3) My spirit needs to be fed with spiritual food—worshiping God, praying without ceasing, praising the Lord with thanksgiving for all things, feeding on His Word by consulting *The Manufacturer's Handbook* at every opportunity.

4) My soul needs to be fed with obedience to every Word that comes from God because it's always hungering and thirsting after righteousness, and trying to feed it with donuts is just a frustration.

5) My body needs to be fed what's good for it and not what's bad for it.

6) IF I will keep my spirit properly fed, and IF I will keep my soul nourished with what it needs, and IF I will keep my body fed with what's good for it, God will keep me healthy and RIGHT-SIZED! No more overhang when each appetite is in proper balance with the others. I'll be a whole person instead of a person with a fraction lapping over.

It sounded wonderful—except for the IFs.

"Lord, I believe everything You've told me, but to put it into action, I'm going to need help from You all along the line. Not just Your help to keep my soul and spirit fed, but help to know what physical groceries I ought to eat and what physical groceries I ought not to eat.

"And Lord, knowledge won't be enough. I'll need Your grace to be obedient to leave off what I shouldn't have, and to eat what's good for me whether I like it or not.

"And Lord, well, You know how I am. It seems like it would be good to have a four-point program I could memorize and follow, a concrete plan for getting this understanding into action. You taught me a long time ago that knowledge without practical application, hearing without doing, was worse than a big waste of time.

"And Lord, if You give me a program to follow, You'll have to give me grace to stick to the program, too.

"And Lord, if there's anything else You think I'll need—something I haven't thought of yet—put that in the package too, will You?

"Thanks, Lord."

It seemed I was asking for a lot, but I learned a long time ago that when Jesus said, "*Ask*, and it shall be given unto you," He wasn't kidding. He *meant* for us to ask.

Well, I had asked. The rest was up to Him.

chapter 5

The Flip-Your-Flab-Forever Program

Are you ready for the program Jesus gave me by the Holy Spirit? The program that lost a pound a week for me for thirty-six weeks, the program that brought me to my ideal weight and has been holding me there for over a year now, without struggle or strain? The program that can flip *your* flap forever too?

Here it is, just as the Lord delivered it to me:

Beginning with your next meal and continuing at every meal without interruption for as long as you desire to reach and maintain your ideal weight,

1) Pray, "Lord Jesus, please bless this food and all those You used to prepare

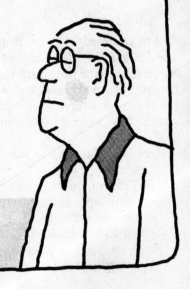

"Lord Jesus, please bless this food and all those You used to prepare it. And now, please match my appetite to my *needs* instead of my *wants*."

it. And now, please match my appetite to my *needs* instead of my *wants*."

2) Eat plenty,
   BUT
3) Stay hungry.
4) Take heavenly vitamins at every meal *and* as often as possible between meals.

That's it? That's it.

I can hear some of you hollering already, "You *can't* mean that's it! That couldn't be all there is to it!" And you sound disappointed because it looks so simple.

"It's just words," you're grumbling. "It'll never work."

I don't blame you for your attitude. It's exactly what *I* thought when He first gave me the program, but being a scientist, and knowing that a *real* one never rejects anything before he tries it, I put the Lord's program to the acid test:

I tried it. On my flab.

I tried it for one week, two weeks, three weeks, four weeks, and every week, the numbers on the scales said I had lost a pound from the week before. Naturally, with results like that, I kept on trying the program, and it kept on working as long as I tried it.

When I had lost thirty-six pounds in thirty-six weeks, I didn't want to lose any more, but I *did* want to maintain my ideal weight without ballooning my way back to fatland. According to the instructions on the program, if I'd stay on it, I'd maintain my ideal weight. That's exactly what happened, and it's still happening.

Only dumbheads argue with results.

"Well, it might have worked for you, but it won't work for me," some diehard insists, and he's perfectly right. I couldn't agree more whole-heartedly. No program will work for anybody who doesn't try it. That's a proven fact.

Pick your corner:

1) You can try the program and keep on trying it and become someone who *used* to be fat, or

2) You can refuse to try the program and become still fatter.

If you've chosen to be among the formerly fat, soon to be free of flab forever, hang around for the rest of the book and I'll tell you how the program works. But first a word to those who are parting company with us along about now, those who are choosing to become fatter still before they're ready to accept God's way in weight control.

If you're a flabbo not quite ready for change, still hiding in the "at least I'm not that bad" shadows of your flabbier friends, don't condemn yourself for lacking the incentive to change. A ball doesn't bounce until it hits bottom. Maybe you *need* to waddle worse before you can stand being trim. Under no conditions should you feel you are a low-grade King's kid just because you overhang in numerous directions. So do bay windows on houses and jowls on basset hounds.

In the fullness of time—which seems to vary from person to person—when you are ready to *accept* the way out instead of merely trying to *comply* with one, come back and join us.

Grudging compliance with a program, against your real druthers, is not recommended. It leads to failure more times than not. Doing something to get the "monkey off your back" is a temporary action that paves the way for a manifold return of the previous yucky condition. When Jesus said that unless a cleansed house contained a new resident the old bad spirit would return with seven others worse than itself, He could have been talking about fatties who take slim-down trips without having their minds renewed by the Spirit of the Lord.

Wait until you know you're hopeless, until you have nothing to offer the program except poverty, inability to help yourself. That's when drunks turn to AA with perfect success—when they've come to the end of their own resources. And the result for them is sobriety for life by putting off the first drink forever, one moment at a time. As a matter of fact, the AA approach fits right into the FFF program, but more of that later.

When you know you're utterly defeated in your efforts to get into a right size, you'll be ready to surrender the old spirit of self-will into the hands of Jesus so He can do as He pleases with you—the temple He lives in. It's the age-old principle of making yourself available to God, who then becomes "God working in you, both to will and to do of His good pleasure." Strangely, His good pleasure becomes better and better—even in our eyes—than anything we had ever planned for ourselves.

The rest of this book is for you who have chosen to flip your flab, becoming "formerly fat" by accepting God's program for reaching and maintaining your ideal weight forever.

chapter 6

Pray

What comes out of your mouth as well as what goes in it is of extreme importance in the Flip Flab Forever program. No, I'm not talking about removing your dentures so you won't be tempted to chomp calories. And I'm not referring to the old Roman vomitariums that let feasters stay slim following the adage, "All that goes down must come up."

I'm talking about the prayer Jesus prescribed for me when I asked Him to give me a method for permanent weight control:

"Lord Jesus, please bless this food and all those You used to prepare it. And now, please match my appetite to my *needs* instead of my *wants*."

Like you, at first I had some reservations about

the prayer Jesus gave me as the first step in the FFF
program (that can stand for Flip Flab Forever or
Former Fatties Free!, whichever fits your fancy). I
don't mean that the words of the prayer were hard to
say, but I thought the prayer was too simple, not
complicated enough for eggheads like me, until He
opened my ears to what I was *really* asking Him
when I prayed it. And then I saw that it was packed
with power to push my paunch right off my bulging
beltline.

First I was to pray that the Lord who fills all things
would bless the food I was about to eat. But did the
food need to be blessed, my educated idiot box
wondered. After all, *I* was the one who needed the
blessing, not the food.

"Don't knock it, Hill. Blessing the food on your
plate is a big order. Do you realize that if I didn't
bless your food before you ate it, it would probably
kill you?"

"*Kill* me, Lord?" Remarks like that didn't do much
to whet my appetite.

"That's right. With all the additives in the food in
your supermarket basket these days to embalm it so
it won't seem stale when you eat it, and with all the
chemicals put on vegetables to make them grow
bigger, faster, and with all the insecticides to kill
bigger and badder bugs, and all the hormones fed to
chickens and cows to beef them up for market in a
hurry, you generally have a whopping load of poison

on your plate when you sit down to eat. If you don't ask Me to bless it, it's your funeral."

Could the Lord be exaggerating a little bit? I hoped so, but in the meantime, instead of eating the next meal, I headed for the library to do a little research.

Nope, He wasn't exaggerating—except maybe to understate the case just a little. Results of my research are given in further detail in chapter seven, but to sum it up, the facts as set forth in all kinds of consumer reports, nutrition books, and newspaper headlines were so gruesome I was glad I had Mark 16:17-18 on my side. Checking to make sure it was still in my *Manufacturer's Handbook*—since it was a life or death matter—I breathed a sigh of relief when I found it there in black and white. (If your Bible is a red-letter edition, you'll find it in red and white, because Jesus is the One who said it.) "These signs shall follow them that believe . . . if they drink any deadly thing it shall not hurt them."

Since a blender can liquefy almost anything, I figured it was safe to assume the verse referred to God's protection against poison foods as well as poison beverages. I had a glory fit right there on the spot. Just think! All the years when I didn't know any better than to eat poisons, the Lord had been protecting me! Now that He was telling me to *ask* Him to bless the food, I was more than glad to do it.

After asking Jesus to bless the food—to make the poison in it nonpoisonous to me—next I was supposed to ask Him to bless all the ones who helped prepare the food. At first I thought He meant just the cook in the kitchen, but then He opened my eyes wider on that too.

Behind the person who burned my toast—my wife or a waitress somewhere—were the men who made the toaster, the clerk who sold the bread, the man who owned the supermarket, the baker who kneaded the dough, the inventor of the machine that sliced and wrapped it, the engineer who kept the power station going to supply electricity for the ovens, the miller who ground the wheat, the farmer who planted it, the rats that didn't eat it, the cat that didn't eat the rat. . . .

It was like the house that Jack built—*everyone* got into the act somehow. The simplest meal involved the preparation of an infinite number of folks. In having me pray for all of the people who helped to prepare my food, the Lord was asking me to pray for practically everyone in the whole world! That was a tall assignment!

"How come I'm supposed to pray for everybody, Lord? My mashed potatoes will turn to cement while they wait."

"Prayer will get your digestive system into shape to handle the groceries, Hill. There's no way you can hold a grudge or resentment against anyone if you're praying for Me to bless them. Your prayer will put you into a right relationship with My people and you'll land on a wavelength of forgiving and rejoicing where there are no ulcers, no colitis, no constipation, no diverticulitis, no heartburn, no nausea. . . . Furthermore, you won't be in danger of eating a single extra mouthful to feed resentment, unforgiveness, or to celebrate a pity party. Instead, as you pray for everybody, you'll be in a perfect position to have the next part of your prayer answered:

"'Please match my appetite to my *needs* instead of my *wants*.'"

Sure enough, as soon as I prayed the prayer, I sensed that the third part of it was on the verge of answering itself. I could almost feel my wants shrinking, coming into harmony with the actual needs of my physical body. With the appetites of my spirit and soul being fed with what was "meat meet" for them, I wouldn't have to shell out as many shekels for meat at the supermarket. For a Scotchman like me, that was good news! I wouldn't have to risk having to pay first-class airfare to get a seat wide enough either.

My appetites were coming into proper balance! I could feel it happen as I prayed!

And I guess here's as good a place as any to let you in on something important I discovered way back near the beginning of my life as a King's kid. (Maybe you know it already, maybe you don't.) Here it is:

Prayer isn't just saying words. Prayer is getting ahold of God, really making two-way contact with Him.

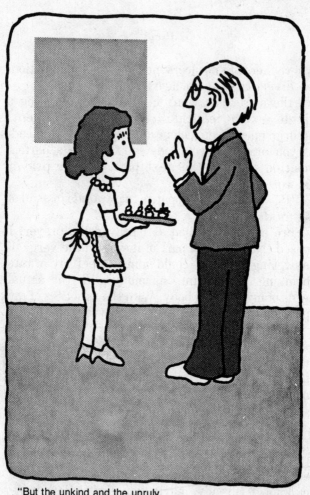

"But the unkind and the unruly,
And the sort who eat unduly,
They must never hope for glory—
Theirs is quite a different story!" (Robert Louis Stevenson).

Pray

Since God is a spirit, you can't reach Him just by stretching out a hand to grab Somebody. The only way to contact spirit is with spirit, and if you haven't been born again (born of the Spirit, that is), it's likely that your efforts to communicate with God have been big fat failures. No wonder.

One night a man named Nicodemus came to talk to Jesus about these things. Their conversation is recorded in chapter three of the Gospel according to John. You can read it and get born again yourself, just as Jesus recommended, and then you can begin to have two-way communication with God. It's better than a CB radio. I tell how I got born again in the first five chapters of my *How to Live Like a King's Kid*. Becoming a King's kid is an absolutely essential prerequisite to having the Flip Your Flab Forever program work for you.

chapter 7

Eat Plenty

"Lord, I see the point of the first step of the FFF program now, but this second one makes about as much sense as putting lead pontoons on a seaplane: Eat Plenty. I always thought the de-blubbering process from slob to sliver could only take place by a method akin to slow starvation."

"You *thought*. That's the trouble, Hill. You're always thinking. Can't you remember that the whole head is sick, just like I said in Isaiah 1:5?"

"Yes, Lord," I told Him, but because my mind was so made up in reverse gear, it took some deliberate listening for me to hear what He was saying in this second step of FFF.

"Eat plenty. Eat plenty. Eat plenty," percolated in my think tank for several days before I could hear that He was *not* saying, "Eat plenty of fattening foods and poison additives and everything else bad for you." Instead, of course, He was trying to get across to me, "Eat plenty of what's *good* for you."

Well, that solved one problem—and introduced another one. I knew what was good *to* my taste buds, of course. I'd known that for years—ice cream of any flavor, cake (especially Black Forest cake), apple pie a la mode (deep-dish preferred, because there was more of it), French fries, biscuits, T-bones, goodies of every description, the sweeter and richer, the better. I had a sneaking suspicion those were the very things responsible for upholstering my frame so plushly, and I didn't suppose the Lord was telling me to eat plenty of *them* and compound my problem. There must be a difference between what was good *to* me (the things I wanted) and what was good *for* me (the things my body needed).

Which was which? The evidence of my senses hadn't proved too helpful in the past. For instance, I'd always been careful to avoid undressed salads, baked fish, green vegetables, and low calorie sweeteners because people who ate such things were always the flabbiest folks around. Leaving them off, I had more room for country-style steak with two helpings of mashed potatoes and gravy and plenty of dessert. But maybe eyeball evidence wasn't reliable.

As a first step in learning what was what, I decided to check *The Manufacturer's Handbook*. When I picked it up, the pages fell open to the Book of Daniel, so I started reading there. The very first chapter was loaded!

It seemed that when the Babylonian King Nebuchadnezzar seized Jerusalem, he asked his chief officer, Ashpenaz, to pick out a few of the best-looking and brightest of the Israelite young men for a special three-year-training-course to fit them for service in the royal court. Ashpenaz was to teach them to read and write the Babylonian language, and while he was at it, he was to give them royal treatment, even to providing them the same food and wine as the king himself enjoyed.

Daniel must have had more sense than I'd have had under the circumstances. Instead of saying, "Oh, boy!" and using the king's orders as an excuse to dive into all the kingly delicacies with gusto, he chose to stick to the dietary laws God had laid down for His people, not to deprive them of goodies, but to insure them of health and long life.

"No thanks," Daniel said to Ashpenaz when he passed the platters groaning with every fattening food you could name. "I'd like just vegetables and water, please, with some whole grains and fruit. No wine, gravy, or apple pie for me—and leave off the meat. Just give me simple fare."

Such a thing was unheard of, and poor Ashy must have thought Daniel had a loose connection in his cranium. Besides that, he was afraid he'd be in permanent trouble with his own head—like maybe having to get along without it after it was chopped off by order of the king—if Daniel's diet made him scrawny. But Daniel talked Ashy into letting him and three friends try the simple food routine for ten days. Then he examined the evidence to see how they looked compared to the young men gorging themselves on the royal diet.

How did it turn out? Well, Danny and his friends looked so great compared to the pasty flab of the other young men that Ashy let them continue choosing their own food for the duration of the training period. Judging from what happened later, their choices had a lot to recommend them:

1) Simple food must be good for sharpening gray matter and upping IQs, because *The Manufacturer's Handbook* says that Danny and his cohorts were ten times smarter than anyone else in the whole kingdom.

2) Simple food must have been good for fireproofing turbans and kimonos, too, according to a picture I remembered seeing in a children's picture Bible— but that's another story. (You can read all about it in the third chapter of Daniel.)

3) Daniel's eating the simple food God prescribed *could* have had something to do with the lions coming down with lockjaw in his presence, a real life or death matter for Daniel. (You can read about that in Daniel, chapter six.)

However you look at it, Daniel's diet, as prescribed

by the Lord, was exactly right for Daniel.

Another newbie that came to my attention in the Book of Daniel is one that seems to have been overlooked by staffers of all the overflowing mental institutions in our country. Did you ever notice how old Nebuchadnezzar got cured of insanity? God put him on a diet of fresh grass for seven years. It's something to think about.

Well, there was so much about food in the Book of Daniel, I turned back to Genesis to take a nutritional tour of the whole *Manufacturer's Handbook*. I haven't finished it yet by a long shot, but I've learned some fascinating things about how it pays to chew plenty of the right food all along—and to *es*chew the no-no food.

Right off to start with, I was reminded that Adam and Eve wouldn't have fallen from grace and dragged the whole human race along with them if they had stuck to the diet God gave them. If Eve had been eating plenty of what the Lord had said was good for food, she'd have turned off the devil's temptation with a simple, "No thanks. I've had plenty to eat already."

And if Esau had been eating plenty all along, he wouldn't have come in so famished from a hunting trip that he paid too high a price for a bowl of stew and regretted it ever after.

If the Israelites had been content with the manna God gave them day by day instead of trying to save some leftovers for midnight snacks, they could have avoided maggots in their garbage. Ugh! And if they had been satisfied with what God gave them—manna in the morning and quail at night—instead of crying for more and more meat, they wouldn't have died from the overdose.

In Leviticus, I found an interesting prescription that, if taken as God had meant it, could have kept us from cholesterol problems forever. He said it so plainly: "This is a lasting ordinance for the generations to come [that's us], wherever you live: You must not eat any fat" (Leviticus 3:17).

And we wouldn't have had to go to the nutritionists to learn that pork's not all that good for King's kids if we had listened when God said that His people weren't to eat the flesh of animals that didn't chew the cud. Pigs are too busy grubbing for more and more groceries ever to chew the same thing twice. Maybe here the Lord was saying that we ought to chew our food more thoroughly too. Seems I've heard twentieth-century doctors recommend that for good digestion.

There was no end to the wholesome nutrition rules in *The Manufacturer's Handbook*. Whole grains fresh out of the fields, fresh fruits, vegetables, honey, milk, no artificial preservatives (the manna bit taught me that), no fat. . . .

If I'd been following His rules all along, I'd never have gotten into such bad shape to start with.

After checking out some of what the Manufacturer had to say about the best fuel for His people, I consulted a few folks with a lot of experience in helping others take off poundage.

"In the Flip Flab Forever program the Lord gave me," I told them, "He said I should eat plenty of what's good for me. Does that make sense to you? Will it work? Does it get results with the flabbos you're shrinking?"

"Yep, it's thoroughly scientific," they nodded, knowing my background. "If you eat plenty of what's good for you, your stomach will be satisfied and you'll be less likely to go overboard at the first whiff of temptation." That was good, and then I learned something even better! The things *The Manufacturer's Handbook* recommended for King's kid ingestion were the very ones successful shrinkers ate! Furthermore, the things God said I should steer clear of were still bad for me, according to modern science. No conflict.

The more I read, the more I saw that God knew where it was at, from the very beginning. I wondered, though, if He ever imagined how many no-nos we'd be eating by the twentieth century. It seemed everybody was building deadlier mouth traps. I learned that a lot of what I had been stuffing into my gullet was working like cyanide, just a little more slowly. He hadn't exaggerated about the poisonous foods at all. Get a load of a few of the more dangerous additives I found out about in *A Consumer's Dictionary:**

Calcium sulfate. Often called Plaster of Paris, this is a fine ingredient in wall plaster, cement, and rat poison. But it's also used in some kinds of white bread, cereal and flour! Could turn you into a real rigor mortis. No thanks, I'm not interested in any more white bread if one of its ingredients could kill the rats in the pantry.

Coal tar derivatives. These have all kinds of fancy names—methyl calicylate, absinthium or wormwood—that one was named for the devil's nephew, no less! Some coal tar derivatives have been proven to cause cancer in laboratory animals, and they are at least highly questionable for human consumption. Others are strong irritants and small amounts can cause severe poisoning that can make you wish you were dead. A dose just a little bit larger can make your wish come true. Still others might not kill you, if you're in pretty good shape to start with, but they'll give you headaches, uncontrollable trembling, and convulsions that would make ordinary DTs look like a study in immobility.

I surely didn't want to eat any coal tar derivatives! That meant I had better lay off some kinds of ice cream, candy, liquor—I'd done that already—baked goods, and certain brands of bottled beverages that were loaded with additives. Would you believe that half a gallon of good old ice cream from the supermarket could contain up to sixty chemical additives I'd be better off without?**

Sodium thiosulfate. It sounded dignified enough to feed royalty, but vets use it to treat ringworm and mange. I didn't know that potatoes were susceptible to these diseases, but they must be because food processors use the same chemical to treat French fries so they won't turn brown. Well, I was glad to learn that I wouldn't get the mange from eating French fries, but I started turning green contemplating the prospects.

Butylated hydroxanisole (BHA) and BHT (butylated hydroxytoluene) are two chemical additives often used in ice cream, processed potatoes, breakfast cereals, baked goods and other desserts, and some shortenings. Being studied by the FDA in the United States, the buty brothers are already banned in foodstuffs in England. Some university research indicates these culprits have damaging effects on brain patterns.

Monosodium glutamate (MSG), used in many products to intensify meat and spice flavorings (it's cheaper than using more meat and more spice), can also intensify headaches, chest pains, and numbness in the appendages. Law prohibits its use in baby foods now, but it can still be used to weaken grownups. People who frequent places featuring Oriental cuisine are likely to come down with a rash of symptoms, collectively labeled "Chinese

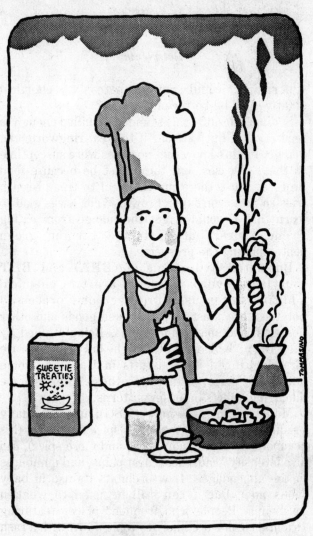

Enriched and fortified, but still poison.

Restaurant Syndrome," and MSG is the culprit.

Diethylstilbestrol is a synthetic estrogen (a hormone) fed to cattle and poultry to fatten them fast for the market. A proven carcinogen, it guarantees that consumers will be fatter corpses sooner. Several European countries already prohibit the use of DES in cattle feed, and it's under further study by the FDA in this country. Meanwhile, it does its deadliest unhampered. How to avoid it? Ease up on meat and chicken unless you can grow your own and grow un-insecticided feed for them. Better yet, eat the grain yourself instead of wasting some of it in growing leather and chicken feathers.

Ficin, an enzyme occurring in the latex of tropical trees, is used to tenderize meat and to remove casings from "skinless" sausages. You can imagine what it does to *your* insides. Highly irritating, to say the least.

Sodium ptoluene sulfochloramine is a real mouthful. You're likely to get some every time you bite into a hunk of processed cheese. Seems to be good for the cheese—but for folks? Watch out! It can cause loss of consciousness, circulatory collapse, and a bill from the funeral parlor. Other chemicals used in processed cheeses are equally scary. The solution? Don't eat them. Stick to natural cheeses.

Parts of aphids, flies, moths, weevils, cereal beetles, and assorted rodent hairs. These may not appeal to you as desirable ingredients in frozen pot pies, but you're sure to have some on your plate and in your system if you buy the supermarket offerings, according to *Consumer Reports.* ** The same publication warns that canned sardines may have unwelcome contamination from feathers—maybe a seagull got too nosey about the canning process? Whatever the label, when you buy processed foods you're sure of paying for some ingredient you'd rather *not* have. But it comes with the package.

White sugar? According to the labels I've read, it appears in almost every processed food on the market. And every nutrition book says it's pure poison, killing God's people right and left. Go ahead and buy sugared cereal for the kiddies—if you want to get rid of 'em legally.

Well, it doesn't take a genius to figure out that most of the poison additives and empty calories that are put in food are added to cater to the lust of the eyes (artificial coloring), the lust of the flesh (hyper flavor to satisfy dulled taste buds), the love of money (manufacturers using cheaper ingredients and masking the fact with chemical pepper-uppers), impatience (already-prepared foods loaded with preservatives so mama can get supper on the table in a hurry without missing her favorite soap operas), or laziness (buying the potatoes already mashed instead of peeling your own).

I got willing to do without the artificial eye appeal and the embalming qualities and the rest of the second best when ı got wıse to what the additives were doing to me! The whole effect made me willing to consider a diet closer to nature. Nutritionists said that would not only be better for me, it would be easier on the bank account. Who could argue with a recommendation like that?

One day the Lord gave me a handy rule of thumb about some of these things. It went like this: "Avoid all things white except as directed. Eat all things green unless specifically prohibited." It was a rule easy to remember. Things pale as death—white bread, white flour, white sugar, ice cream, too much salt, and lard—were likely to lead to Dead Man's Gulp.

As a further guide to directing my appetite toward the things I ought to have ar.d killing it for the no-nos, I ran across this yes and no list:***

1) Don't eat anything containing refined (white) sugar in any form. That included corn syrup, sucrose, dextrose, lactose, corn sugar, or any of the other aliases for refined sugar. Do eat products containing unrefined sweeteners, such as honey, unrefined molasses, pure maple syrup, and unrefined sugar.

2) Don't eat any product containing refined (white) flour. Do eat products made with 100% whole grain flour.

3) Don't eat processed fruits or vegetables. Chances are they've been mutilated in the process of being canned, jarred, dehydrated, or frozen. Do eat

fresh fruits and vegetables—home grown if available—in as nearly their original form as possible. Highly recommended are potatoes in their skins, apples with the peel, fresh melons, peaches off the tree, peanuts fresh from the shell.

4) Avoid soft drinks except those you make yourself at home, using fresh fruits or herb teas and natural sweeteners. The store-bought variety is full of poison sugar, poison coloring, water polluted with carbonic acid, and bankrupting tendencies.

5) Avoid store-bought sauces such as ketchup, salad dressing, steak sauce, and barbecue sauce. Make your own—they'll be cheaper, tastier, and better for you.

6) Avoid prepared snack foods. They're loaded with additives, empty calories, and other ingredients that will damage your health, sex appeal, and bank account. Try munching on carrots, celery, radishes, and green peppers until you've flipped your flab. Then you can add nuts, seeds, popcorn, whole-grain crackers, sesame seed cookies made with honey, dates, and peanut-butter balls rolled in coconut fresh off the monkey tree.

Other sources said I should think about eating far less meat than had been my custom, switching to fish and poultry or even to legumes and other protein-rich meat substitutes. That way I'd avoid a lot of flab-building fat and improve my cholesterol standing. I'd already noted that Adam and Eve didn't have to eat meat in the perfect beginning of things and we probably won't be eating it in the New Jerusalem where known carnivores like lions will be lying down peacefully with the lambs who were formerly their lunchmeat. Getting into the habit of less meat earthside—or becoming altogether vegetarian—could be good boot-camp preparation for a heavenly hereafter.

After I had learned some of what was behind the prohibitions and recommendations for my digestive system, I began deliberately to seek out and eat the things that were good for me. To my surprise, I *liked* them! Made me feel clean, somehow. Taller. And in eating plenty of the right things, my whole health situation began to improve, to say nothing of my conscience. Some of the old cravings, so full of grease and empty sugar calories, began to look repulsive to me. I could see that the Lord was reprograming my appetite, making me desire the things that were "of good report." It was no longer a matter of the old self-denial that had created a compulsion for the very things that were killing me, but a growing desire not to corrupt my body—His temple—with deadly poison and have to suffer the consequences.****

"Eat plenty of what's good for you!"

"Lord, I'm ready. And I'm even going to do a little figuring to see if I can add a row or two to my garden so I can actually count on a few meals where I won't have to "plead the blood" over every forkful.

I sensed a fringe benefit on the horizon—the extra plowing, planting, cultivating, weeding, and harvesting would be good exercise for me too.

A Consumer's Dictionary of Food Additives, by Ruth Winter (New York: Crown Publishers, 1978).

**The Supermarket Handbook: Access to Whole Foods*, by Nikki and David Goldbeck (New York: New American Library, 1976), p. 309.

***Adapted, in part from *Everything You've Always Wanted to Know About Nutrition*, by David Reuben, M.D. (New York: Simon and Schuster, 1978).

****Consult Appendix I for some reading material that can help you in reprograming your appetite for food fit for King's kids. Appendix II contains a few recipes to change your cooking habits from no-nos to right-ons!

chapter 8

Hunger

"Lord, You've just persuaded me, against my preliminary better judgment, that I'm to eat plenty, and now You're telling me to stay hungry." I didn't tell Him to make up His mind, but I halfway wondered if I had heard wrong.

Once again, I had raised a sick-head mental block He had to overcome before He could get His wisdom down into my top ten inches.

As He does so often, He resorted to His printed Word, knowing I've finally reached the place where I'm likely to accept that without too much of a fuss. I guess that's why He took me to a concordance for the next step. There it was, *hunger* as a verb, with nine entries in my abridged concordance. That ought to be enough to clue me in to what He was driving at with

His "Stay hungry."

The first reference, back in the Old Testament in Deuteronomy, was a real blockbuster:

> And he humbled thee, and suffered thee to
> *hunger*, and fed thee with manna . . . that
> he might make thee know that man doth not
> live by bread only, but by every word that
> proceedeth out the mouth of the Lord.
> (Deuteronomy 8:3)

He was telling me that I was supposed to be hungry, not for things on the breakfast table, but for what He provided—the Bread of Heaven!

And get a load of what followed in the very next verse:

> Thy raiment waxed not old upon thee,
> neither did thy foot swell, these forty years.
> (Deuteronomy 8:4)

Even I know that if a man can wear the same suit for forty years, and if his feet don't swell when he makes like a pedestrian for all that time, his weight is well under control. That sounded so good, I just had to read on, and was I ever glad I did! Look at the next promise I found:

> For the Lord thy God bringeth thee into a

good land, a land of brooks of water . . . A
land of wheat, and barley, and vines, and fig
trees, and pomegranates; a land of oil olive,
and honey; A land wherein thou shalt eat
bread without scarceness, thou shalt not
lack any thing in it. (Deuteronomy 8:7-9)

What a mouthful the Lord provided when His
people had hungered for a while! And it was all food
that was good for them! Pretty right-on for an Old
Testament statement about the advantages of
hungering now and then. Made me want to know
what the New Testament had to say.

I remembered that Jesus said, "Blessed are they
which do hunger and thirst after righteousness, for
they shall be filled." He didn't say with *what* they
would be filled, but when I checked the *Amplified
Bible*, I found this wording:

Blessed and fortunate and happy and
spiritually prosperous . . . are those who
hunger and thirst for righteousness
(uprightness and right standing with God),
for they shall be COMPLETELY
SATISFIED! (Matthew 5:6)

I'd always before equated hunger with total
misery, but Jesus was saying that the right *kind* of
hunger could lead to total satisfaction. I was in favor

of that!

And on the subject of satisfaction, the Lord dumped another goodie my way in Deuteronomy 8:10 where I read, "When you have eaten and are satisfied, praise the Lord your God . . ." (NIV).

Maybe that would help keep the whole digestive system in order—praising the Lord every time I ate Complaining about food, on the other hand, seemed to be a dangerous thing to do. According to Moses, one time when the Israelites had been griping about their grub, "There is no bread! .   And we detest this miserable food" (Numbers 21:5 NIV), a lot of them died off with snakebite. When the people repented, "Moses made a bronze snake and put it up on a pole" (Numbers 21:8 NIV) so anyone who looked at it would live and not die. Being reminded of the snakebites that came to those who grumbled about groceries, I resolved to eat what was set before me without being too critical.

Well, searching the scriptures about hunger got better and better as I went along. The first thing I knew, it was suppertime, and I had skipped lunch without even missing it because I was so satisfied with sloshing around in the Word, storing it down in my gizzard.

Staying hungry—for righteousness, for the Bread of Life, the Word that proceeds out of the mouth of God—is joy unspeakable and full of glory for King's kids.

If that's what His "Stay hungry" was talking about, it was one of the most satisfying things in the world.

As I pondered that, another thought came, along these lines. If I was dissatisfied when I was too fat, then it was logical that hungering to be the right size—setting that as one of my priorities, kind of a goal to work toward—could be helpful.

A woman I know—let's call her Draggy Dora because that's what she used to be—told me that when she started hungering to be the right size, she became impressed that she needed to get some exercise every day. But when?

Dora's days were fully scheduled already, she figured. Finding a niche for exercise looked impossible, and to tell the truth, her preferences ran to more sedentary activities. But Dora was well acquainted with the Lord and knew that settling impossible situations was His specialty, so she asked Him about it.

"Lord," she prayed one day, "I keep getting the feeling that You want me to get a move on, but it's impossible for me to find the time for it." She recited her calendar to Him as if He couldn't read it for Himself.

"If You want me to exercise, You're going to have to figure out where and when and let me in on it."

Dora was hoping He wouldn't find a place, and would just excuse her from the requirement, but she had done a dangerous thing—she had put the

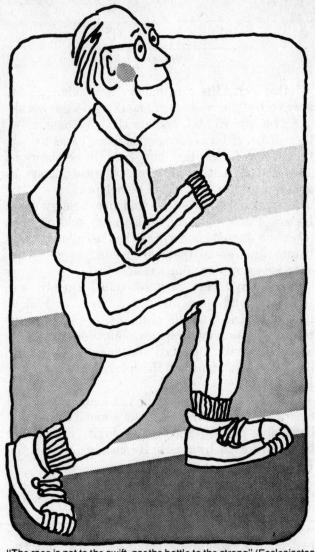

"The race is not to the swift, nor the battle to the strong" (Ecclesiastes 9:11 RSV).

problem in the Lord's hands.

Lo and behold! The Lord showed Dora half an hour she didn't know she had! Furthermore, it was at a perfect time not to interfere with the rest of her day but to improve it.

At eight o'clock every morning, Dora's children left for school and her husband took off for work. A married daughter who lived half a mile away often dropped in for a little chat about the same time. Dora would pour her a cup of coffee, shove her a donut, and they'd sit and visit.

"There's your exercise time, Dora. Down with the donuts, full speed ahead. You and Matilda can talk while you walk—every day in your former fattening time. You'll still have your mother-daughter fellowship—minus the donuts that have been settling like a permanently inflated life preserver around your waist—and the walk will have long-term benefits. In a year, it can make a twelve-pound difference in your weight all by itself. To say nothing of the difference in your outlook that thirty minutes' worth of fresh air can make. It'll be good for your daughter too."

"But Lord, how about bad weather? Surely you don't want us to walk in the rain?"

"In Arizona already? Besides, who do you think invented raincoats, overshoes, and umbrellas? A walk in the spring rain, if you can find some, is one of the very special treats I have for King's kids."

"But how about when it's thundering and lightning, Lord? Surely you don't want me to be electrocuted!"

Dora was the most persistent diehard of my acquaintance—next to me.

"So okay. Once every thousand years, it'll lightning between eight and eight-thirty in the morning. That day, you and your daughter can take turns riding the indoor exercycle that's been gathering dust in a corner of the attic. Clean it off and bring it down so you'll be ready for that inclement weather. I wouldn't even mind if you sat on it and pedaled some morning while you're dipping into My Word. . . ."

Dora was finally persuaded—and so was I—that the Lord can show us time for exercise if we ask Him. And Dora's report after she'd been at it for a couple of months?

"Yes, I've reached my right size now, and I'm convinced God will keep me there on the FFF program whether I walk or not. But I wouldn't give up the walking for anything! Matilda and I have found it's one of the best parts of our day—makes all the rest of it go better. And since we both have our Bible time with the Lord before breakfast, we have plenty to talk about with each other, sharing what the Lord has shared with us. It's funny—but we're both so glad I used to be fat. . . ."

What Dora's experience said to me was that any

flabbo who was serious about getting his earthly temple in shape could find time to exercise if he'd only ask the Lord to show him.

While I was thinking along these lines, the Lord reminded me of the scripture where Paul was talking about keeping his eyes on Jesus and running toward his goal with patience. I looked it up to refresh my memory, and again I hit pay dirt, a scripture that was thoroughly relevant to de-blubbering. *The Manufacturer's Handbook* put it this way:

> Wherefore seeing we also are compassed about with so great a cloud of witnesses, let us lay aside every weight, and the sin which doth so easily beset us, and let us run with patience the race that is set before us, Looking unto Jesus the author and finisher of our faith. . . . (Hebrews 12:1-2)

I don't know what that verse says to you, but that day the Lord used it as a real incentive and faith-builder in my life. It was as if Paul was saying he was a flabbo too and encouraging himself and me with these words: "Since so many people are looking at us, Hill, let's get rid of our weight—lay aside this flab—and the stuffing ourselves which comes so easy but isn't God's best for us. Let's head toward our right size patiently (no overnight slim-down that will prove strictly temporary), looking to Jesus who can make it possible for us to get there."

I'd always suspected that Paul was a little on the paunchy side. He was such a perfectionist, it'd have been hard for him *not* to have been an alky or a food-a-holic, one or the other. I know, because I've been there—both places.

Well, you can take that interpretation or leave it, but it seems that every time I turn to *The Manufacturer's Handbook*, whether it's about eating plenty, staying hungry, or trying to find out what I should eat, He has something to say on the subject. And it always matched up with what the "experts" told me too.

For instance, in checking with the paunch-pruning specialists about staying hungry, I found they were in agreement with what God had told me. One of the de-blubbering experts affirmed that along with eating plenty of what was good for me, I should stay hungry—by which he meant that I should quit eating before I felt quite full.

It sounded like agony to me, but he said I wouldn't find it so bad once I'd tried it.

"Fullness of time is a biblical principle, all right," he told me, "but it also seems to have something to do with this weight business. You see, it takes awhile for the blood sugar to build up after you've taken in some grub. If you eat enough, instead of too much, and then just wait a little while, you'll find your appetite satisfied that didn't seem to be satisfied at first. It just requires a little time for the carcass to know it's been fed when it's been overstuffed so long its sensors have burned out."

I tried his recommendation the next meal, leaving second helpings in the serving bowl instead of throwing them down my gullet without even taking a breather.

You know, the guy was right! Half an hour after lunch I felt like I'd had enough to eat after all and would probably last five hours till supper without expiring from starvation.

There were all kinds of new tricks the Lord was teaching me as I followed His plan. And now, there was only one of the four major program steps left to go.

chapter 9

Vite!

"Take heavenly vitamins at every meal and as often as possible between meals."

What in the world could that mean? Heavenly vitamins? Who had ever heard of such a thing? Not me. Furthermore, I didn't think God had heard of them either.

Just on the outside chance that I might have missed something, I checked the biggest concordance I could find. It skipped right from *visiting* to *vocation*, not a vitamin in sight. Looked like a dead end, but the Lord has never specialized in leading me down blind alleys. He always has *something* for me in everything He says, if I can just get hold of it. What could it be here? Vitamins? Heavenly vitamins?

Earthly vitamins of the garden variety were necessary to bodily health, I knew. Practically every package I looked at in the kitchen cupboard said something like, "Provides the following percentages of the Minimum Daily Requirement of Vitamins A—XYZ as established by the powers that be." The MDR, I knew, was something you had to have for a healthy body.

Could there be such a thing as a MDR of heavenly vitamins—whatever they were—for spiritual health? And could they be related in some way to the success of the FFF program?

Health. That was a good word. I tried it in the concordance that had let me down about vitamins. Pay dirt! Plenty of references.

The first one said that Joseph's father was in good health. I was glad for old Jake, but the information didn't seem particularly relevant to my search.

The second reference had Joab wondering if his brother was healthy. I hoped so, but again, no connection to FFF that I knew of.

The third and fourth references were the Psalmist praising God for being the "health of his countenance," whatever that meant. Sounded like a divine remedy for pimples, a problem I left behind me more than fifty years ago.

The next reference was to a benediction I'd heard a lot. Interesting, but not what I was after. It was getting discouraging. Maybe I was following a wrong lead. But the next entry in the concordance leaped out at me: "It shall be health to thy navel!"

Bullseye! Right on target! The lard around my navel was where it was at! Whatever would bring health to my navel was bound to be a heavenly vitamin. "Thy kingdom come to my navel," I heard myself praying as I turned the pages of *The Manufacturer's Handbook* in record time and made myself start reading the chapter from the beginning so I wouldn't get anything out of context:

> My son [it was plainly addressed to a King's kid—me] forget not my law; but let thine heart keep my commandments: For length of days, and long life, and peace, shall they add to thee. Let not mercy and truth forsake thee: bind them about thy neck; write them upon the table of thine heart: So shalt thou find favour and good understanding in the sight of God and man. Trust in the Lord with all thine heart; and lean not unto thine own understanding. In all thy ways acknowledge him, and he shall direct they paths. Be not wise in thine own eyes, fear the Lord, and depart from evil. *It shall be health to thy navel*, and marrow to thy bones. (Proverbs 3:1-8)

Heavenly vitamins! Remembering and keeping

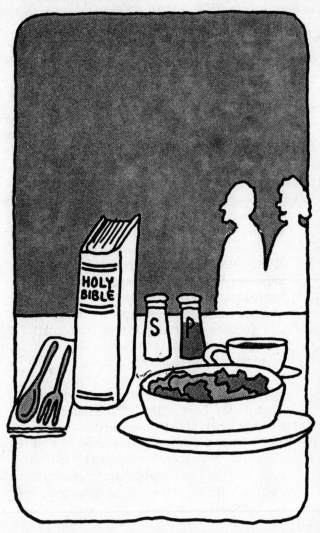

"Heavenly vitamins, to be taken at every meal."

His law, being merciful and truthful, knowing His Word and doing it, acknowledging Him and not being wise in my own eyes, fearing and honoring Him, departing from evil. . . . All these were heavenly vitamins, guaranteed to keep my navel base healthy. No more too-fatness if I hung in there with God's Word.

The next reference confirmed what I had just learned. Get a load of it:

> My son [Hey! That was me again, a King's kid!], attend to my words; consent and submit to my sayings. Let them not depart from your sight; keep them in the center of your heart. For they are life to those who find them, healing and health to all their flesh. (Proverbs 4:20-22 TAB)

His Words, His sayings would be health to *all* my flesh, not just to my navel! Heavenly vitamins! The Word of God! To be taken at every meal!

His laws and statutes were sweeter than honey and the honeycomb, I remembered from a song I'd helped to sing at lots of CFO camps. Maybe I should have scripture for dessert—and for an appetizer too!

It sounded like it was worth trying. That night I took one of my Bibles and put it on our kitchen table alongside the salt and pepper shakers and the African violet my wife had parked there.

"Heavenly vitamins," I told her when she raised her eyebrows at me. "To be taken at every meal."

Maybe she understood why, maybe she didn't, but the Bible's still there and mama and I sample some of it every time we sit down to eat. It's made a difference in more than just my size.

It would take a whole shelf of books to hold all the Lord began to show us when we started taking heavenly vitamins at every meal. Appendix III has a lengthy list of heavenly vitamins to give you a start at compiling your own.

Altogether, the scriptures are the most mind-renewing, flab-flipping agents I know anything about.

Celia, a woman who took the FFF plan seriously— a hefty sixty pounds of her *needed* it— told me her life style usually prevented her doing any scripture reading at mealtimes, but she modified the plan so she could use it anyhow.

"Six months ago, I set my alarm for an hour early every day," she said. "I'd get downstairs before it was light, while everyone else in the house was still sleeping, and I'd do my Bible reading and praying then. That way, I had plenty of heavenly vitamins inside me that I could chew on at mealtime."

Well, that sounded okay to me, but I wasn't sure how practical it was. There was one way to find out.

"Did it work?" I asked her.

She grinned like a Cheshire cat with a canary inside

her. "Thirty down and goal to go," she said. "I'm well on my way out of blimphood and headed toward slim sisterhood, thanks to the Lord."

If that approach worked for her, there's no reason you can't try it for yourself.

Lots of people complain they have trouble finding enough time for Bible reading. Some solve it like Celia did, getting up early enough to spend as much time feeding her spirit as she'd spend later feeding her body—an equal time deal. One gal I know uses a daily Bible study guide to keep her reading at a pace that will take her through the whole Bible every year.

Some time ago I became aware that I didn't have as much time as I wanted to really soak in the Word, so I purchased the New Testament in cassette-tape form. That way I could feed on it while driving my car, and at odd times during the day. With tapes, you can get steeped in the Word of Life while you're doing household chores, pulling weeds in the garden, preparing dinner, or soaking in the tub. (If you don't have a set of Bible tapes, write me at P.O. Box 8655, Baltimore, Maryland 21240, and I'll send details about my favorite New Testament version. Don't forget to enclose a self-addressed stamped envelope.)

Soak up His Word whenever and wherever you can. That way you'll gradually build up a supply of the Word down inside you, and it'll be ready to come forth to meet every need of your life.

Vitaminize. Vite! It's no accident that the abbreviation the Lord gave me for this chapter means *lively* in music. *Vite!* We are lively—full of life—when we follow the Lord's plan for flipping flab forever—or doing anything else worth doing.

chapter 10

How Flipping Flab Works for Good

Pray, Eat Plenty, Hunger, and Vite! There you have the FFF program as the Lord gave it to me. You see the value of each part and how it all fits together. That's all you have to know to put it into action, flipping flab forever from *your* frame. Nothing else is required.

But the Lord always does above all we could ask or think or even dream of. And He didn't just give me the basic plan, explain it, and then leave me on my own. He provided continual help for every step, and He'll do the same thing for you. Furthermore, He'll keep providing new incentives, new bits of growth as you hang in there with His Word, taking your heavenly vitamins as they are prescribed. And likely you'll find, as I have, that the program doesn't just

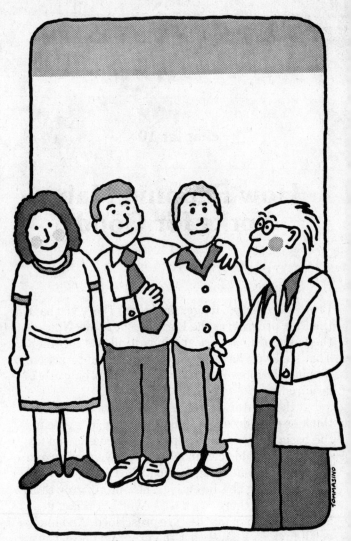

King's Kids are conquerors!

flip your flab forever, it does something to the rest of you. It seems to be a part of an overall purifying plan, helping to get rid of all the wrinkles, spots, and blemishes that make us less than perfect vessels for the priceless treasure that we hold when we become King's kids. And as we get cleaned up, we begin to think more in terms of Jesus' coming back again to claim His bride, the church, and we want to live our lives to His glory instead of to suit our own druthers. As a matter of fact, He works the whole FFF plan—which is a plan for wholeness—for such good in the lives of former flabbos that they become glad they were fat enough to be interested in the program!

If you've read my other books, you know something about how the Lord can't use any of us in ministry to others until we have tribulated through something ourselves. Now if you've been flabbo and you've started slimming down on the FFF program, you won't be able to hide your progress under a bushel. Pagans are going to notice the change in your dimensions.

"How come I haven't been seeing so much of you lately?" they're likely to ask. "You look wonderful—what there is of you. I'd like to lose some weight myself. Mind letting me in on the secret?"

One day I received a letter from a flabbo who asked the question in a poetic manner.

Dear Mr. Hill, please pray for me,
    I weigh two hundred eight.
    I've lost control and can't resist
    The goodies on my plate.

I yearn for pies, I drool for cake—
    My cravings never cease.
    I diet, but my frame expands
    From "fat" to "most obese."

My husband calls me "chubby"
    And sleeps down in the den;
    My best girlfriend just laughs at me,
    She weighs one hundred ten.

I say, "I won't eat pizza!"
    And swear I won't drink beer;
    I promise to give up hot rolls;
    And I am most sincere!

But temptation's all about me and
    My vows are so much blab;
    So tell me, Mr. Harold Hill,
    How did you flip *your* flab?

                Sincerely,
                Myrtle Fatlips

    Questioners are entitled to answers, and if you handle their inquiries just right—looking to the Lord for guidance—you can chalk up a new King's kid every time.

    "Lord, is *that* why You've allowed so many King's

kids to get so blubbery?" I asked Him one day. "So that when they slimmed down following Your plan, the pagan world would notice and get harvested for the Kingdom?"

He didn't answer me directly, but I thought I heard a slight chuckle from on high. The next time I had my hands on a phone book with yellow pages, I looked up the subject "Reducing and Weight Control Services." There were health spas of every nationality, TOPS Clubs (to take off pounds sensibly), Weight Watchers, Figure Salons, Diet Workshops, Diet, Discipline, and Discovery groups, Overeaters Anonymous. . . . You name it, there was an outfit by that name—everything except Flab Flippers.

Many of the organizations were good ones, I found out, with sound programs for slow, steady, permanent weight loss based on good nutrition. A few even had Bible study and prayer as a part of their programs. Some of the outfits were second best, offering instant weight loss for the impatient, with medications that promised practically painless miracles overnight, shrinking flab with drugs dangerous to your health and to the peace and safety of those about you. It was obvious that the plans that didn't involve a whole new approach, repro-gramming of appetites, offered only temporary relief from the widespread problem.

But all of the groups, whether they knew it or not,

were using one basic biblical principle—fellowship—
because they met weekly for weigh-in, lectures, sharing of setbacks and victories, low-calorie recipes, and
encouragement of one another (another biblical principle). Some provided more frequent meetings for
tape-measuring and exercise programs.

Should you join such a group? Ask the Lord. If
you're just dying to "join something," He might tell
you there's no harm in following the FFF program in
the midst of the fellowship of an already established
group of fellow strugglers. God just might want to
use you in such a group to point the way for some
other flabbos to receive Jesus and know the joy of
FFF His way. King's kids are called to be witnesses
wherever they are.

The sound nutritional programs of such outfits as
Weight Watchers could be very helpful to you, giving
you a right eating program; the help-one-another
approach of Overeaters Anonymous has a lot to offer
too. But you don't have to pay initiation fees and
weekly dues to some fellowship to flip your flab with
someone who understands the problem. You could
get together for weigh-in and encouragement with
someone in your own family. One bulgy husband and
his chubbier wife decided to flip their flab forever
family style. They taped a sheet of yellow tablet
paper to the bathroom wall, right above the scales.
Each records his/her weight there every day—no

cheating—and one of them charts it on a graph stuck on the front of the refrigerator! The eyeball evidence is that they're shrinking steadily together as they grow in the Lord.

A plumpish woman who happens to have a skinny husband made a prayer pact with a chubby chum down the block. They call their duo the Flab Flippers Club—what else? At any time of the day or night when compulsion strikes and backsliding threatens, the about-to-be-a-victim telephones the other and asks for help in postponing that first bite (or sip) of lard-building potion for one more twenty-four-hour period. In taking such action, they're latching onto the principle used with great success by Alcoholics Anonymous, which can claim more than a million former problem drinkers who have postponed that "first one" for periods up to forty years. The chubbies' hubbies are rejoicing as they watch their wives shrink.

"But what if my chubby chum doesn't answer the phone?" one not-that-badder asked me after a seminar one day.

"Simple solution," the Lord directed me to answer her, instead of silently consigning her to the hosts not-yet-ready-for-help. Then He let me elucidate: "In cases when you think you're all alone in your temptation and can't contact another human being, try praying for yourself, something immediate like this:

Lord, I'm about to succumb to that first bite. Please do something about it or I'll fall back into my former slavery to that goodie. Lord, if You can't handle this compulsion, that makes two of us, because I can't handle it either. But if You *can* do something about it, please do it right now. Thank You. Amen."

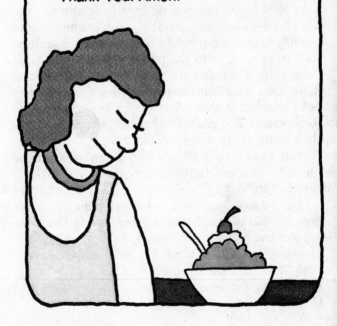

"Lord, I'm about to succumb to that first bite. Please do something about it or I'll fall back into my former slavery to that goodie. Lord, if You can't handle this compulsion, that makes two of us, because I can't handle it either. But if You *can* do something about it, please do it right now. Thank You. Amen."

This prayer didn't work for the not-that-badder because she didn't try it. But it has worked for me and for thousands of other folks about to lose the will-power battle with the bottle, so it's bound to do likewise for flab fighters who are serious enough about it to humble themselves and pray.

It's as true for fatties as it is for alkies that it's easier to *stay* off the forbidden fruit than it is to *get* off it again after the first bite or sip. Instead of "This first bite won't count," the truth is that the first bite is the only one that can get you in trouble. Avoid that one, and you've won the ball game.

Plumpies who band together to help one another with their overstuffed condition seem to have an edge on those who try the solo route. That's the Lord's plan, I figure, because He never designed us to be isolated persons but to work together in teams of at least two people where big problems have to be dealt with. Even Jesus sent His disciples out two by two—for a reason.

Looking at the advantages of teamwork as spelled out in *The Manufacturer's Handbook* can be mighty persuasive. Look at this goodie for instance:

> Two are better than one; because they have
> a good reward for their labour. For if they
> fall, the one will lift up his fellow: but woe to
> him that is alone when he falleth; for he hath
> not another to help him up. . . . and a
> *threefold* cord is not quickly broken.
> (Ecclesiastes 4:9-10, 12)

Two sounded good, and a trio sounded even better
for depounding. Five? Listen to this!

> Five of you shall chase an hundred [that's
> twenty pounds apiece], and an hundred of
> you shall put ten thousand to flight [most of
> us don't have a hundred to spare].
> (Leviticus 26:8)

It sounds like "Band together, boys!" would be a
good battlecry for blimpos who want to be
deflated. If you've been trying the FFF plan with
negligible results, and the flab still hangs in great
gloppy gobs bearing a strong resemblance to a hound
dog's ears hanging off your wretched torso, take a
hint from these scriptures and get together with a
fellow sufferer. As you intercede for one another,
both of you may start to shrink—to the glory of God.

Ministering God's blessings to others is part of His plan. As we become channels for His grace to other folks, our souls are opened wide to the free flow of the love of God which blesses us with all *we* need on its way through.

"How come so many Spirit-filled Christians are bulging out all over the place?" I asked the Lord one day after noticing the overstuffed audience at a Full Gospel Business Men's Regional Convention. "I haven't seen any statistics on it, but the evidence is that King's kids are more likely to be bursting at the seams than the run-of-the-mill pagan world. I've even heard 'em quote scripture on it. 'Who loves the Lord, the Lord makes fat,' they spout at me and say it comes from Proverbs somewhere."

"People have always tried to blame Me for their sins," He seemed to say. "But I never gave anybody a body and told him to abuse it with gluttony. Even *you* know that, Hill. And your senses are giving you right evidence, for once. My people *are* too fat. The reason? These are the folks who used to take part in the rat race. They were tearing around like chickens with their heads cut off, killing themselves with nicotine, alcohol, chasing other men's wives—or husbands. After they met Me, they settled down. The vices that used to take so much time and energy are gone from their lives, and they just sit around reading My Word and go to banquets where they praise Me and lovingly pass refreshments to one

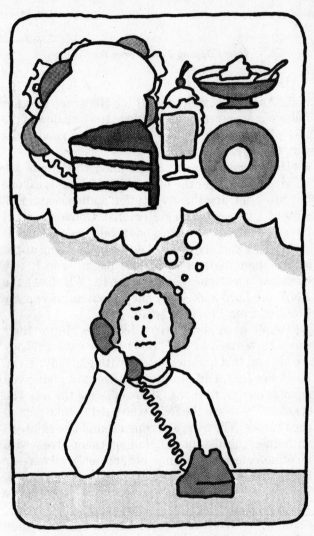

Fortify your faith by phoning a flab-flipping friend.

another.

"They have been so accepting of themselves, knowing I have forgiven them for everything, that they haven't condemned themselves for eating everything in sight. It was kind of like they had given up everything illegal and immoral and so the only things that were left to them were fattening. They kept quoting, 'There is therefore now no condemnation,' and making more apple pie for themselves and the brethren. Hospitality overflowed everywhere. . . .

"*But* a new thing is happening now, Hill. The fat has reached a peak, and My people are waking up to the fact that it isn't a good witness for them to be bulging out all over. They're beginning to want to look presentable—for Me. They want to be walking advertisements for My ability to give them self-control instead of puffing examples of self-indulgence. They want to *be* perfect—and *look* perfect—for My sake.

"That's why I've given you the FFF plan, Hill. Not just to get you in shape, but so you can share it with those who are ready for it.

"Spread it around, Hill. Spread it around."

I told Him I would do it. And you can help too. Begin now. The fatter you are, the better. Call your fat friends. Invite them over for lunch. Put the right kind of food on the table. Ask them if they'd like to join you in flipping their flab forever, following Jesus' plan.

They'll be glad you did. So will you. And so will I. Best of all, so will He.

Appendix I

Publications for Plumpies

A few books and other publications to whet your appetite for what's right—and to tell you where and how to get it:

> *The Supermarket Handbook: Access to Whole Foods*, by Nikki and David Goldbeck, (New York: New American Library, 1976). A Signet book, available for $1.95, this publication gives you a complete course in the fine art of label-reading, teaches you to recognize the unnecessary additives that raise prices and may be harmful to your health, and provides you with a listing of the best quality foods by brand name. It's chockful of useful

information about nutritious, whole, and natural foods, and tried-and-true recipes, proving that right-eating can be fun! Contains helpful bibliographies, including one of cookbooks "to guide you along."

Consumer Reports, published by Consumers Union, Mt. Vernon, New York. A monthly magazine with frequent reports on good and bad foodstuffs.

Organic Gardening and Farming, published by Rodale Press, Emmaus, Pennsylvania. A monthly magazine which keeps you warned about what's bad for you and helps you grow what's good for you. "The Pesticides in the Food You Buy," in the March 1979 issue is an eye-opener that might turn you overnight into an organic gardener.

Prevention, published by Rodale Press, Emmaus, Pennsylvania. A monthly magazine that keeps you on your toes about good nutrition, exercise, and related subjects designed to keep the body in top-notch condition.

Let's Eat Right and Keep Fit, by Adelle Davis, (New York: New American Library, 1970). A Signet book that provides a thorough know-how on nutrition.

Appendix II

Food for Flab-Flippers

Some thoughts on food for flab-flippers:

Simple food is good, and right cooking doesn't have to be complicated. As a matter of fact, the easier something is to prepare, the better it is likely to be for you! Less cooking, more vitamins, generally speaking.

Here are two easy-to-fix meals that will be good for you:

1) Lay freshly filleted fish (catch it yourself if you can, otherwise buy it at a fish market) skin side down in a shallow pan. Put in a 350° oven for twenty to thirty minutes (cooking time depends on size of fish; you can tell that it's done when it loses the translucent look and when it's easily flaked with a fork), season to taste and serve. Lots of people think

they won't like fish if it isn't heavily breaded with cornmeal and fried to within an inch of its life. Many are agreeably surprised when they try baked fish. It's better than ever! And infinitely better for them.

If you put a couple of well-scrubbed baking potatoes (red "new potatoes" are especially good baked) in the oven three-quarters of an hour before the fish, you'll be two-thirds of the way to a perfectly nutritious, no-bother feast that fits calorie requirements for slimmers. The other third? Try grating cabbage, carrots, and green pepper together (a blender makes quick work of it), then toss with a "dressing" made with vinegar sweetened with a spoonful of natural honey.

Eat plenty—but stay hungry—and while you're waiting for your blood sugar to tell you you're satisfied, take your heavenly vitamins as prescribed.

2) Another no-work meal if you're still eating poultry—maybe grandma has a chicken coop and you can talk her out of a fryer that hasn't been hormoned into fatland—goes like this:

Salt and pepper a small fryer inside and out. Stick the liver in the empty insides, and put the chicken, legs up, in a shallow pan in a 350° degree oven. Put the chicken neck, gizzard, and heart (if your chicken happened to have one) in a small pan of water and let it simmer while the chicken bakes.

An hour later, turn the chicken over to brown its back and put some brown rice on to cook (follow instructions on the package). When you're ready to set the table, cook green beans crisply tender (freshly picked if you have a garden in season, home canned or frozen if you don't) with a chopped onion, freshly ground pepper, and a sprinkling of basil instead of the hog fat you *had* to use for seasoning everything until you noticed you were starting to fatten like a hog yourself.

Put chicken on a heated platter and make the gravy. Don't worry. It'll be legal for dieters if you make it right. Pour giblet juice into baking pan and scrape up all browned-on bits. Pour liquid into tall container and skim off fat as it rises—all of it. Blend a small amount of the fat-free liquid with whole wheat flour to make a smooth paste, add to liquid and boil for tasty "greaseless gravy."

Pour homemade tomato juice in glasses for an appetizer. Rice and snap beans ready? I thought so. Sit down and enjoy another simply good-for-you meal. If you're still flabbo, eat the chicken breast instead of the drumsticks and leave the skin on your plate. Who gets the liver? Not enough to divide, so you'll have to draw straws.

Both of these meals are so simple, a child can fix them, except for maybe mom's touch on the gravy.

For a good basic eating plan while you're shrinking, find a friend who belongs to Weight Watchers and ask to look over their food plan. It doesn't leave out anything you need for good health, and it provides a satisfying assortment of allowable foods so you won't get bored to death with what you're supposed to eat. Best of all, their plan eliminates calorie counting for the shrinker—the organization has pre-counted everything for you. A real plus. And if you don't know that a handful of salted peanuts or potato chips will wreck the course of flab-flippers who want to get on with it, stop by your local public library and check out a nutrition book with a calorie chart and bone up on the subject.

A good motto from *The Manufacturer's Handbook* is " 'Everything is permissible for me'—but not everything is beneficial. . . . I will not be mastered by anything" (1 Corinthians 6:12 NIV). It's hard not to be mastered by a peanut or a potato chip unless you choose to leave them off. The choice is always yours, and ignorance of the simple facts can lead to second best—which is what got you to flabland in the first place.

For snacktime, successful shrinkers head for the cookie jar—which is kept in the refrigerator, filled with carrots, celery, apples, and cucumbers. Crave something a little more exotic? Don't lust after a double hot fudge sundae. Any slob can have one of them, and probably does, frequently. Treat yourself to a handful of sprouted sunflower seeds toasted in a moderate oven to semi-crispness. Good? Beats ambrosia.

Appendix II

Eating right—for flab-flipping and for good health forever after—doesn't have to be dull. You can begin an adventure into right cooking with *The Rodale Cookbook* and *Rodale's Naturally Great Foods Cookbook*, both by Nancy Albright and published by the Rodale Press of Emmaus, Pennsylvania.

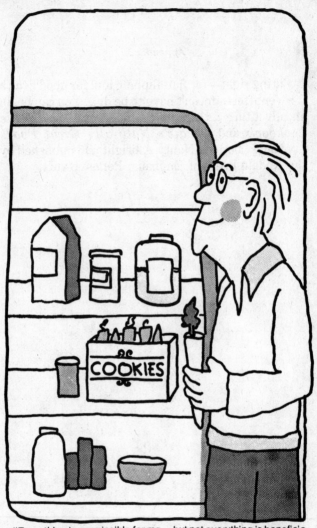

"Everything is permissible for me—but not everything is beneficial"
(1 Corinthians 6:12 NIV).

Appendix III

Heavenly Vitamins

R_X: "Take heavenly vitamins at every meal and as often as possible between meals."

The Manufacturer's Handbook is full of chewable heavenly vitamins, but here are a few "extra-choice ones," P, G, E, T, and F, to get you started on filling in the rest of the alphabet for yourself. Each morning for the next two weeks, choose one vitamin from two or more categories and chew on them all day. Right away, you'll find benefits accruing for yourself, the persons for whom you pray, and the partners with whom you pray.

You may leave these vitamins in the book (they don't require refrigeration). Use them like a "promise box" on your table.

Remember, these are just to get you started.

You'll be adding your own as you explore His Word.

Here they are, a few vitamins P, G, E, T, and F.
Spelled out, they stand for:

Power-Packed Promises
Grace for God's Glory
Examples of Encouragement
Temptation Trompers
Fruitful Fellowshipers

Heavenly Vitamin P— Power-Packed Promises

---

1 Faithful is he that calleth you, who also will do it. (1 Thessalonians 5:24)

---

2 Being confident of this very thing, that he which hath begun a good work in you will perform it until the day of Jesus Christ. (Philippians 1:6)

---

3 [Not in your own strength] for it is God Who is all the while effectually at work in you—energizing and creating in you the power and desire—both to will and to work for His good pleasure and satisfaction and delight. (Philippians 2:13 TAB)

4 Now we have received, not the spirit of the world, but the spirit which is of God; that we might know the things that are freely given to us of God. (1 Corinthians 2:12)

5 But the Spirit produces love, joy, peace, patience, kindness, goodness, faithfulness, humility, and self-control. (Galatians 5:22 TEV)

6 For the kingdom of God is not meat and drink; but righteousness, and peace, and joy in the Holy Ghost. (Romans 14:17)

7 With men it is impossible, but not with God: for with God all things are possible. (Mark 10:27)

8 If ye abide in me, and my words abide in you, ye shall ask what ye will, and it shall be done unto you. (John 15:7)

9 The eyes of all mankind look up to you for help; you give them their food as they need it. You constantly satisfy the hunger and thirst of every living thing. (Psalm 145:15 TLB)

10 And Jesus said unto them, I am the bread of life: he that cometh to me shall never hunger;

and he that believeth on me shall never thirst. (John 6:35)

11 Man shall not live by bread alone, but by every word that proceedeth out of the mouth of God. (Matthew 4:4)

12 I will instruct you (says the Lord) and guide you along the best pathway for your life; I will advise you and watch your progress. (Psalm 32:8 TLB)

13 Thou wilt keep him in perfect peace, whose mind is stayed on thee: because he trusteth in thee. (Isaiah 26:3)

14 Nay, in all these things we are more than conquerors through him that loved us. (Romans 8:37)

Heavenly Vitamin G—Grace for God's Glory

---

1 For the Lord God is a sun and shield: the Lord will give grace and glory: no good thing will he withhold from them that walk uprightly. (Psalm 84:11)

---

2 And of his fulness have all we received, and grace for grace. For the law was given by Moses, but grace and truth came by Jesus Christ. (John 1:16-17)

---

3 For God has revealed his grace for the salvation of all mankind. That grace instructs us to give up ungodly living and worldly passions, and to live self-controlled, upright and godly lives in

this world. (Titus 2:11-12 TEV)

---

4 It is good to receive inner strength from God's grace, and not by obeying rules about foods; those who obey these rules have not been helped by them. (Hebrews 13:9 TEV)

---

5 And if by grace, then is it no more of works: otherwise grace is no more grace. But if it be of works, then it is no more grace: otherwise work is no more work. (Romans 11:6)

---

6 For sin shall not have dominion over you: for ye are not under the law, but under grace. (Romans 6:14)

---

7 But unto every one of us is given grace according to the measure of the gift of Christ. (Ephesians 4:7)

---

8 And he said unto me, My grace is sufficient for thee: for my strength is made perfect in weakness. Most gladly therefore will I rather glory in my infirmities, that the power of Christ may rest upon me. (2 Corinthians 12:9)

---

9 For God resisteth the proud, and giveth

grace to the humble. (1 Peter 5:5)

---

10 But grow in grace, and in the knowledge of our Lord and Saviour Jesus Christ. (2 Peter 3:18)

---

11 But he giveth more grace. Wherefore he saith, God resisteth the proud, but giveth grace unto the humble. (James 4:6)

---

12 Be strong in the grace that is in Christ Jesus. (2 Timothy 2:1)

---

13 Let us therefore come boldly unto the throne of grace, that we may obtain mercy, and find grace to help in time of need. (Hebrews 4:16)

---

14 The grace of the Lord Jesus Christ, and the love of God and the communion of the Holy Ghost, be with you all. (2 Corinthians 13:14)

Heavenly Vitamin E Examples of Encouragement

1 Therefore if any man be in Christ, he is a new creature: old things are passed away; behold, all things are become new. (2 Corinthians 5:17)

2 When I pray, you answer me, and encourage me by giving me the strength I need. (Psalm 138:3 TLB)

3 God is faithful, by whom ye were called unto the fellowship of his son Jesus Christ our Lord. (1 Corinthians 1:9)

4 The Lord will perfect that which concerneth

me: thy mercy, O Lord, endureth for ever. (Psalm 138:8)

5 Great is his faithfulness; his lovingkindness begins afresh each day. (Lamentations 3:23 TLB)

6 Seek your happiness in the Lord and he will give you your heart's desire. (Psalm 37:4 TEV)

7 In everything you do, put God first, and he will direct you and crown your efforts with success. (Proverbs 3:6 TLB)

8 Don't be frightened by the size of the task, for the Lord my God is with you; He will not forsake you. He will see to it that everything is finished correctly. (1 Chronicles 28:20 TLB)

9 I publicly praise the Lord for keeping me from slipping and falling. (Psalm 26:12 TLB)

10 For whatsoever is born of God overcometh the world. (1 John 5:4)

11 Tell everyone who is discouraged, "Be strong and don't be afraid! God is coming to your rescue." (Isaiah 35:4 TEV)

12 I can do all things through Christ which strengtheneth me. (Philippians 4:13)

---

13 But thanks be to God, which giveth us the victory through our Lord Jesus Christ. (1 Corinthians 15:57)

---

14 And let us not get tired of doing what is right, for after a while we will reap a harvest of blessing if we don't get discouraged and give up. (Galatians 6:9 TLB)

---

15 Now no chastening for the present seemeth to be joyous, but grievous: nevertheless afterward it yieldeth the peaceable fruit of righteousness unto them which are exercised thereby. (Hebrews 12:11)

Heavenly Vitamin T—Temptation Trompers

1 Why spend your money on foodstuffs that don't give you strength? Why pay for groceries that don't do you any good? Listen and I'll tell you where to get good food that fattens up the soul! (Isaiah 55:2 TLB)

2 Labour not for the meat which perisheth, but for that meat which endureth unto everlasting life, which the Son of man shall give unto you: for him hath God the Father sealed. (John 6:27)

3 Let us examine our ways and turn back to the Lord. (Lamentations 3:40 TEV)

4 If ye then be risen with Christ, seek those

things which are above, where Christ
sitteth on the right hand of God. Set your
affection on things above, not on things on
the earth. (Colossians 3:1-2)

5 For we fix our attention not on things that
are seen, but on things that are unseen. (2
Corinthians 4:18 TEV)

6 What? know ye not that your body is the
temple of the Holy Ghost which is in you,
which ye have of God, and ye are not your
own? For ye are bought with a price:
therefore glorify God in your body, and in
your spirit, which are God's. (1 Corinthians
6:19-20)

7 And so, dear brothers, I plead with you to
give your bodies to God. Let them be a
living sacrifice, holy—the kind he can
accept. . . . Don't copy the behavior and
customs of this world, but be a new and
different person with a fresh newness in all
you do and think. Then you will learn from
your own experience how his ways will
really satisfy you. (Romans 12:1-2 TLB)

8 Blessed is the man that endureth
temptation: for when he is tried, he shall

receive the crown of life, which the Lord hath promised to them that love him. Let no man say when he is tempted, I am tempted of God: for God cannot be tempted with evil, neither tempteth he any man: But every man is tempted when he is drawn away of his own lust, and enticed. (James 1:12-14)

9 There hath no temptation taken you but such as is common to man: but God is faithful, who will not suffer you to be tempted above that ye are able; but will with the temptation also make a way to escape, that ye may be able to bear it. (1 Corinthians 10:13)

10 And now he can help those who are tempted, because he himself was tempted and suffered. (Hebrews 2:18 TEV)

11 Greater is he that is in you than he that is in the world. (1 John 4:4)

12 Submit yourselves therefore to God. Resist the devil, and he will flee from you. (James 4:7)

13 Fear thou not; for I am with thee: be not dismayed; for I am thy God: I will

strengthen thee; yea, I will help thee; yea, I will uphold thee with the right hand of my righteousness. (Isaiah 41:10)

---

14 Last of all I want to remind you that your strength must come from the Lord's mighty power within you. (Ephesians 6:10 TLB)

Heavenly Vitamin F— Fruitful Fellowshipers

1 And one standing alone can be detached and defeated, but two can stand back-to-back and conquer; three is even better, for a triple-braided cord is not easily broken. (Ecclesiastes 4:12 TLB)

2 Again I say unto you, That if two of you shall agree on earth as touching any thing that they shall ask, it shall be done for them of my Father which is in heaven. For where two or three are gathered together in my name, there am I in the midst of them. (Matthew 18:19-20)

3 But if we walk in the light, as he is in the

light, we have fellowship one with another, and the blood of Jesus Christ his Son cleanseth us from all sin. (1 John 1:7)

---

4 Blessed be God, even the Father of our Lord Jesus Christ, the Father of mercies, and the God of all comfort; Who comforteth us in all our tribulation, that we may be able to comfort them which are in any trouble, by the comfort wherewith we ourselves are comforted of God. (2 Corinthians 1:3-4)

---

5 Let us be concerned for one another, to help one another to show love and to do good. Let us not give up the habit of meeting together, as some are doing. Instead, let us encourage one another all the more, since you see that the Day of the Lord is coming nearer. (Hebrews 10:24-25 TEV)

---

6 But exhort one another daily, while it is called To day; lest any of you be hardened through the deceitfulness of sin. (Hebrews 3:13)

---

7 Bear ye one another's burdens, and so fulfil the law of Christ. (Galatians 6:2)

---

8 Confess your faults one to another, and

pray for one another, that ye may be healed. (James 5:16)

9 We then that are strong ought to bear the infirmities of the weak, and not to please ourselves. Let every one of us please his neighbour for his good to edification. (Romans 15:1-2)

10 Look not every man on his own things, but every man also on the things of others. (Philippians 2:4)

11 For as we have many members in one body, and all members have not the same office: So we, being many, are one body in Christ, and every one members one of another. (Romans 12:4-5)

12 A new commandment I give unto you, That ye love one another; as I have loved you, that ye also love one another. By this shall all men know that ye are my disciples, if ye have love one to another. (John 13:34-35)

13 Finally, be ye all of one mind, having compassion one of another; love as brethren, be pitiful, be courteous. (1 Peter 3:8)

14 Behold, how good and how pleasant it is for brethren to dwell together in unity! (Psalm 133:1)

Appendix IV

Questions and Answers

God's promise "Ask and it shall be given unto you" obviously includes "Ask for answers and you will get them." This appendix is made up of some of the questions flabbies have asked me lately, along with the answers the Lord has directed. If you have any questions that aren't included, and you want answers, write me in care of Logos International, 201 Church Street, Plainfield, New Jersey 07060, and we'll see what can be done. Be sure to include a self-addressed stamped envelope for reply.

Q What about fasting as a way to lose weight?
A Anything as drastic as prolonged fasting should be undertaken only under careful medical supervision. Fasting can lead to a starvation

syndrome called *anorexia nervosa* that terminates not only the flab but the patient himself, bones and all. So beware!

Furthermore, some doctors prescribe fasting as an effective treatment for underweight patients, so watch out again! Abstinence from food for a period of time *can* lead to rapid weight gain *above* the original level when the fast is ended.

There is, however, an important exception to the rule that fasts should be undertaken only upon medical advice. There is the highly recommended—for everybody—King's kid fast that goes like this:

Once a month, enter into a thirty-day fast from all complaining, fault-finding, nit-picking, and criticism as you begin to praise God in, for, and in spite of all earthly appearances. Since God inhabits the praises of His people, the fuller you are of God, the less likely you are to pack in too much of anything else.

Q I've started your flab-flipping plan, and I'm shrinking, but not fast enough to suit me. What do you recommend?

A Patience. Slow losing is better than fast losing. A gradual, steady weight loss gives time for new right-eating habits to be firmly established. Furthermore, it gives an opportunity for your skin to shrink to fit the new you without the danger that you'll trip over loose folds caused by too rapid evacuation of fatty tissue.

Resist the temptation to be impatient, because impatience leads to discouragement and discouragement leads to giving up just when victory is in sight. Fast streamlining and fast frustration seems to go hand in hand. Fullness of time takes time, and so does permanent flab-flipping.

Q How about diet soft drinks?

A If you're interested in giving the mortuary an increase in business, drink all the diet soft drinks you want. The more, the better. If however, you're more interested in a long and fruitful life, leave them off entirely.

First of all, artificial sweeteners are poison. Notice the sign warning you about products containing saccharin the next time you go to the grocery store. It's the law that they have to tell you saccharin may kill you, but they're left free to sell it to you anyhow. Praise God that you're still free *not* to buy it.

Furthermore, the bubble-producing material in diet soft drinks, or in the other kind, is another poison—carbon dioxide gas. Some of it escapes as a "whoosh" when you pull the pop-top or open the lid. The rest, dissolved in the liquid, orchestrates dissonant burps and squeaky stomach rumbles deep within while you're sitting in church.

You think soft drinks pep you up? Think again. And if you won't take my word for it, try a convincing experiment. Concentrate all the carbon dioxide gas in a buck's worth of carbonated soft drinks (wholesale) in an airtight bag. Stick your head inside, tie a string around your neck so none of the gas will escape, and lie still for thirty minutes. After the thirty minutes, you won't have to try to lie still; it'll be automatic—your only option.

The plain fact is that every time you imbibe a bottle of carbonated chemicals you're imbibing the equivalent of a quantity of human exhalation and some highly questionable chemicals dissolved in water you could get free at any public drinking fountain.

The water by itself can invigorate you. Add the noxious elements and you're headed for exhaustion.

Q I get so hungry between lunch and supper. Is it okay for flab-flippers to snack between meals?

A Of course. But only if you snack on low-calorie good-for-you foods—fresh fruits and vegetables—not on calorie-loaded peanuts or additived-to-death ice cream and cookies. Again, read up on good nutrition in the wide variety of publications available on the subject.

Appendix IV

Q I tried your flab-flipping plan and prayed the prayer at every meal for weeks. But yesterday, the scales flew apart when I stepped on 'em. What did I do wrong?

A Probably everything you did between meals. Write down all the "I won't count this one little nibble" mouthfuls of grease-laden "innocent" snacks—potato chips, peanuts, and candy bars washed down with soda pop—you've ingested *without* praying between meals and you'll have writers' cramp *and* an accurate description of the culprit. Wipe him out and you'll begin to see progress in the right direction.

Q Obesity runs in my family. For generations, all members have been broader than they were tall. Is my case hopeless? What do you recommend?

A Broader than you are tall? For starters, you might try slithering around on your side for a while to get a heightened view of the landscape. That could encourage you to be the first in your family to climb down from the food wagon and onto the self-honesty level of admitting you are powerless over your flab. When you tell that to Jesus and ask Him to take over, you'll begin to see a huge difference!

Hopeless? There's no such word among King's kids.

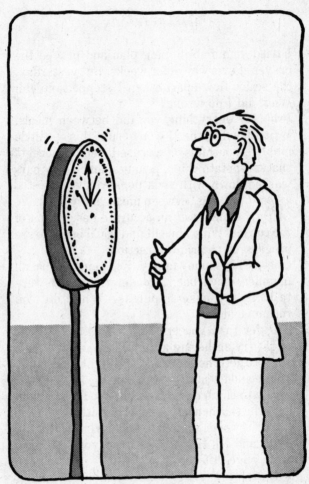

"Let us lay aside every weight, and the sin which doth so easily beset us . . . Looking unto Jesus, the author and finisher of our faith" (Hebrews 12:1).

King's Kid
HAROLD HILL

"P.S. By the way, King's Kids, have you been reading my King's Kids Korner Kolumn in the *Logos Journal*? If so, why haven't I heard from you? If not, send in your subscription TODAY on the form below and I'll see you in the next issue!"

Please send me a subscription to the Logos Journal with Harold Hill's King's Kid Korner Kolumn. I have enclosed payment.

I want to subscribe for:

☐ 1 Year $6.69   ☐ 2 Years $12.38   ☐ 3 Years $18.07

Name _____

Address _____

City_____State_____Zip _____

Mail this coupon and check to:
LOGOS JOURNAL, 201 CHURCH ST., PLAINFIELD, N.J. 07060
OUTSIDE THE UNITED STATES PLEASE ADD $2.00 EXTRA PER YEAR.

Bestselling Books Available at Your Bookseller or use Convenient Tear-Out Order Form
— Quality soft-cover books —

———— **Ask Me, Lord, I Want to Say Yes**— $1.95
Rosalind Rinker—author of Prayer—
Conversing With God

———— **Bible and the Bermuda Triangle**—   2.50
Don Tanner and George Johnson
(over 350,000 sold)

———— **Big Three Mountain-Movers**—   1.95
Jim Bakker—host of PTL-TV

———— **Challenging Counterfeit**—Raphael Gasson   1.95
Exposé on spiritualism

———— **Child of Satan—Child of God**—   2.25
Susan Atkins with Bob Slosser
Charles Manson's woman meets God in prison

———— **Daughter of Destiny**—Kathryn Kuhlman—   1.95
Jamie Buckingham—the most famous woman
preacher—her life—her story

———— **China: A New Day**—Stanley Mooneyham,   2.50
President of World Vision, gives inside
information and how China fits into your future

———— **Day the Dollar Dies**—Willard Cantelon   1.95
Your money's future—what to do to protect it

———— **Do Yourself a Favor: Love Your Wife**   1.95
H. Page Williams (300,000 sold)—the best book
on husband and wife relationships

———— **How to Flip Your Flab—Forever**—
Harold Hill   2.50
The final-diet book

———— **Healing Light**—Agnes Sanford   1.95
Over thirty-six printings

Total this side $ ————————

(more on other side)

**Ask your bookseller for these other bestsellers
(or use this convenient tear-out order form)**

_____ **Thanks Lord, I Needed That!**—Charlene $2.50
Potterbaum—a housewife's practical view on life
(national bestseller)

_____ **Prison to Praise**—Merlin Carothers   2.50
(over 2 million sold)

_____ **Blueprint for Raising a Child**—Mike   3.95
Phillips—every parent's book

_____ **Worth of a Woman**—Iverna Tompkins   2.95
Teaches women their real worth

_____ **Clap Your Hands!**—Larry Tomczak   2.95
A young Catholic finds his faith

_____ **Total Preparation for Childbirth**—Cher   3.95
Randall—acknowledged as a must for future parents

_____ **Victory on Praise Mountain**—NEW!   2.50
Merlin Carothers—the best since Prison to Praise

_____ **Closer Than My Shadow**—Diane Hanny   3.95
A Christian meditation for youth

_____ **People's Temple—People's Tomb**—   2.25
Phil Kerns and Doug Wead
The real story of Jim Jones' cult—
A national bestseller made into a movie

_____ **Holy Spirit and You**—Dennis and Rita   3.95
Bennett   The bestselling book on the
charismatic experience—over 300,000 sold

Total $_____

If unavailable at local bookstores, order through:
LIF BOOKS — Box 191, Plainfield, NJ 07061

Please enclose payment—Sorry, no C.O.D.s—Add 50¢ for
first book, 35¢ for each additional book for postage and
handling

Name _____

Address _____

City _____ State _____ ZIP _____